OKANAGAN UNIVERSITY COLLEGE LIBRARY

P9-EJI-860

# VICTIMS OF CRUELTY

RC 552 .P67 E27 2000
Eckberg, Maryanna,
Victims of cruelty :

## DATE DUE

| | |
|---|---|
| APR 17 2003 | |
| NOV 2 8 2003 | |
| Edmonton Public<br>due Jan 5/05 | |
| | |
| | |
| | |
| | |
| | |
| | |
| | |
| | |
| | |
| | |
| | |
| | |
| | |

BRODART                                    Cat. No. 23-221

# VICTIMS OF CRUELTY

## SOMATIC PSYCHOTHERAPY
## IN THE TREATMENT OF
## POSTTRAUMATIC STRESS DISORDER

———— ·◦· ————

# MARYANNA ECKBERG

Foreword by

### PETER LEVINE

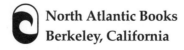

**North Atlantic Books**
**Berkeley, California**

*Victims of Cruelty: Somatic Psychotherapy in the Treatment of Posttraumatic Stress Disorder*

Copyright © 2000 by Maryanna Eckberg. All rights reserved. No portion of this book, except for brief review, may be reproduced in any form—electronic, mechanical, photocopying, or recording— without prior written permission of the publisher. For information, contact North Atlantic Books. Printed in the United States of America

Published by North Atlantic Books
P.O. Box 12327
Berkeley, California 94712

Distributed to the book trade by Publishers Group West

Cover Art by Sara Isabel Rodriquez González
Author Photograph by Ed Bock
Cover and book design by Jan Camp

*Victims of Cruelty: Somatic Psychotherapy in the Treatment of Posttraumatic Stress Disorder* is sponsored by the Society for the Study of Native Arts and Sciences, a nonprofit educational corporation whose goals are to develop an educational and crosscultural perspective linking various scientific, social, and artistic fields; to nurture a holistic view of the arts, sciences, humanities, and healing; and to publish and distribute literature on the relationship of mind, body, and nature.

**Library of Congress Cataloging-in-Publication Data:**
Eckberg, Maryanna, 1938-1999.
  Victims of cruelty: somatic psychotherapy in the treatment of posttraumatic stress disorder / Maryanna Eckberg.
     p. ; cm.
  Includes bibliographical references.
  ISBN 1-55643-353-0 (alk. paper)
  1. Posttraumatic stress disorder—Treatment. 2. Bioenergetic psychotherapy. 3. Mind and body therapies. 4. Torture. 5. Somatoform disorders—Treatment. I. Title.
  [DNLM: 1. Stress Disorders, Post-Traumatic—therapy. 2. Psychotherapy.
3. Somatoform Disorders—therapy. 4. Stress Disorders, Post-Traumatic—psychology. 5. Torture.
  WM 170 E19v 2000]
  RC552.P67 E27 2000
  616.85'21—dc21

                                                                    CPI
                                                                    00-030525

*To my son, Erik, and my daughter, Kristin,
who have brought so much joy into my life.
To survivors everywhere, who have looked horror
in the face and have lived to tell their stories.*

# Table of Contents

## Chapter Three
### TRANSFERENCE AND SOCIETAL TRAUMA

## Chapter Four
### A PSYCHOLOGIST IN EL SALVADOR: PART ONE

## Chapter Five
### A PSYCHOLOGIST IN EL SALVADOR: PART TWO

## Chapter Six
### COLLEEN'S STORY: SURVIVOR OF A NEAR FATAL ACCIDENT

## Chapter Seven
### EDITH'S STORY: A SURVIVOR OF POLITICAL TORTURE

# Acknowledgements

——— ⚜ ———

My heartfelt thanks to my friend and colleague, John Conger, Ph.D., who encouraged me to write and who carefully edited this book. Without his inspiration this book would not have been written. I am extremely grateful to my psychotherapist, Jay Feldman, M.D., who not only "hung in there" with me through very difficult times, but had the courage and persistence to insist that I integrate the horror of my own past. I feel deeply indebted to my dear friend and colleague, Sylvia Conant, R.N., M.N., C.N.S., who gave so generously of her time to do the body-oriented psychotherapeutic work with me, contributing greatly to my healing and, through this experience, to my knowledge of this work. I thank my partner, Peter White, M.S., for his constancy in supporting me emotionally and technologically (solving computer problems) and for contributing his excellent editing skills. For her input into this book and her friendship, my heartfelt thanks to Laura deFreitas, M.A. Special appreciation to my friend and colleague, Judy Bell, M.A., for her conscientious reading of and important comments about the manuscript. I feel much gratitude to my friend and colleague, Carol Bandini, Ph.D., for her careful reading of the manuscript and for her thoughtful feedback. For their continuous stimulation of my thinking in this area by their challenging questions and intense interest, special thanks to my students in the somatics program at the California Institute of Integral Studies, at Clement Street Counseling Center, and at the Healing Center for Survivors of Political Torture. My appreciation to my friend and colleague, Peter Levine, Ph.D., for his unique contribution to the understanding of trauma, which helped so much to consolidate my thinking in this area. I give thanks and due respect to the legacy of Wilhelm Reich, M.D., whose original and creative contributions to somatic psychology and psychotherapy have yet to be fully recognized. To Bessel van der Kolk, M.D., I am grateful for his cutting-edge research on trauma and for integrating much of the work done by other investigators.

# Foreword

———— ·⦿· ————

Maryanna Eckberg leaves us with a precious legacy, a labor of love in the alleviation of suffering. I have known Maryanna for about fifteen years—first as my student and client; and then later in a collegial relationship as therapist, teacher and healer. She worked deeply with me and with others in healing her own profound trauma. She shares this personal case history generously along with several other informative cases adding to the vitality of the book.

Maryanna understood deep trauma. She brings to light, in this significant volume, her years of study and treatment with body oriented psychotherapy. She ties together developmental, analytical, interpersonal, somatic and social-cultural understandings of trauma. She does this with unassuming theoretical clarity and understated clinical brilliance.

Maryanna describes a truly integrative approach to healing deep wounds, whether the traumatic event was the violence of rape, sexual abuse, torture, an auto accident, electroshock treatment or invasive medical procedures and surgery. She shows with clear conceptual understanding and carefully documented case demonstration how energetic approaches that utilize the living, feeling, "knowing" body can help to heal the breach in consciousness triggered by these differing forms of trauma. She does this by integrating the work of Wilhelm Reich, in the form of *Bioenergetic* therapy, the emerging neuro-biological understanding of trauma as advanced by Bessel van der Kolk and his colleagues, and the ethologicaly based *Somatic Experiencing* approach for which she was my student. In making this integration of body, brain, mind and soul in the formation, perpetuation and healing of traumatic shock she contributes to and advances the field. In addition, Maryanna shows how an integrative somatic approach can help heal the deepest and cruel forms of human suffering. She does this in part from her unique experience of working in Central America with victims of pervasive violence and political torture. But she also shows how so many of us are effected by deep states of traumatic shock and how they/we can be healed.

Sadly, she did not get to see the publication of her book; she died shortly after its completion. When I spoke to Maryanna from Europe, I promised to see that her book was published and was pleased that North Atlantic Books took on this valuable project. She expressed to me the deep peace and acceptance she had of her impending death. She also shared her sadness that she would not see the flowering of body oriented approaches in the healing of trauma. Maryanna expressed regret that she would not live to see this renaissance in the healing of trauma through the body. In the form of her book, posthumously published, she certainly joins fully in an emerging paradigm which is changing the course of the contemporary understanding of trauma and its treatment. Join in this adventure, read and be enriched.

PETER A. LEVINE

Foundation for Human Enrichment
Lyons, Colorado

# Introduction

For many years I have been working as a body-oriented psychotherapist with people suffering from trauma, sufferers unable to find comfort in traditional psychotherapy. They include people from El Salvador who were tortured, raped, had their families murdered before their eyes, and also people who have been traumatized growing up in the United States in apparently normal families. The trauma I write about is not only an individual matter, but is the result, as well, of the dark tides manifested when entire societies are traumatized. Thus, I write in this book about El Salvador and torture victims but also describe a survivor of a near fatal bicycle accident. Although I see many people traumatized by accidents and medical procedures, the vast majority of my clients are victims of abuse perpetrated by fellow human beings. I do not subscribe to the theory that everyone is capable of perpetrating abuse on others. For myself, I have decided that evil is very banal. Those who commit inhuman acts generally appear normal. They live ordinary lives within the norms of society. How they differ from those who could not perpetrate abuse on others is not readily visible. I am convinced that they lack the courage to face themselves. At some level they have separated themselves from their own humanity.

My intention in writing this book has been to bring together the traditional world of research and clinical observation in traumatology with the newer world of body-oriented psychotherapy. A bridge between the two worlds seems to be missing. The body is hardly ever mentioned in the numerous books and conferences offered on trauma. Information from research and from the traditional clinical world is likewise ignored in the body-oriented world. Yet the research and clinical observation from the traditional world leads consistently to the same place: "traumatic events are encoded and expressed as somatosensory experience." The world of body-oriented psychotherapy speaks to somatosensory experience.

Recent research in neuroscience and psychoneuroimmunology has provided evidence of the unity of mind-body functioning. Research and clinical data stress emphatically that trauma has a tremendous impact on the body and on how victims experience their bodies. The logical conclusion is that the body plays an essential role in the healing of trauma. However, while those of us in the world of somatic psycho-therapy are convinced by our experience of the significance of the body in the healing of trauma, solid research on somatic interventions in the treatment of symptoms of posttraumatic stress disorder is largely nonexistent. This book was originally conceived out of a feeling of frustration that two worlds that need each other seem to ignore each other.

I entered the traditional world of psychology in 1960 when I returned to the university to complete my undergraduate studies. I then began a graduate program in psychology, and in 1967 I completed my Ph.D. in child and adult clinical psychology.

Shock trauma was rarely addressed directly until the early 1980s. Trauma was being addressed in the Veterans Administration hospitals, where important work with Vietnam veterans was taking place. Yet, for the most part these small pockets of work with shock trauma victims remained isolated from the mainstream. Gradually the impact of having lived through an event outside the realm of normal human experience began to be recognized within the psychological world. Several developments contributed to this. One was the women's movement, in which children's welfare became an important issue. As a result of the feminist movement it became much more difficult to dissociate the serious and extensive problems of child abuse and the abuse of women from our societal consciousness. The traumatic effects of abuse in the seventies began to be recognized and acknowledged. Additionally, work in the area of substance abuse was exposing the very high correlation between experiencing traumatic events, especially abuse, and addiction to drugs. This relationship has become even more apparent in recent years. Work with Vietnam vets was yielding important information about how traumatic events continue to live in-side a person long after the actual experiences have occurred. The *DSM-III* diagnosis of posttraumatic stress disorder evolved out of this important work with veterans. Finally, the Chowchilla kidnapping in Chowchilla, California, in 1976, underlined the tendency to minimize the effects of traumatic experiences. Twenty-six children, five to fifteen years old, had been taken hostage and imprisoned for thirty hours in an underground vault. After they were rescued, they were examined by a doctor and a psychiatrist who declared them to be suffering no ill effects. Eight months later San Francisco psychiatrist Lenore Terr began a follow-up study. She found serious long-term effects in the children, the families, and the whole community (Terr, 1979, 1983).

I was introduced to the world of somatic psychotherapy in 1973 during a month long training in gestalt therapy. In 1975 I began bioenergetic therapy, and I also entered a training program in bioenergetics with the Minnesota Society for Bioenergetic Analysis, associated with the International Institute for Bioenergetic Analysis. Simultaneously, I met Stanley Keleman in Berkeley, California, and started a ten-year process of making two to three trips a year to Berkeley to attend his institutes. I began to sample the many forms of hands-on body work available, including acupuncture, osteopathy, and chiropractic. In 1979 I became a certified bioenergetic therapist, and in 1982 I became a member of the faculty of the International Institute for Bioenergetic Analysis. In 1988 I met Peter Levine, whose in-depth understanding of the body and trauma expanded my knowledge considerably.

Over the years, working with someone on a body level has become so much a part of my being that it is difficult to imagine working without this knowledge. Even though some clients are unable to make a real commitment to work on a body level because it is too threatening to them, I am still seeing through the eyes of a body-oriented psychotherapist, and I am making small interventions on a body level. As will be revealed in my own case history, somatic work played a crucial role in my own process of healing.

My interest in trauma grew in the 1980s as more and more clients with traumatic histories sought treatment from me. At about the same time the details of my personal traumatic past began creeping into my consciousness, revealing themselves to a mind reluctant to acknowledge them. Since then I have worked with many torture survivors, survivors of childhood abuse, and survivors of other forms of trauma. My quest to learn as much as possible about the effects of traumatic experiences on one's psyche and soma and about how trauma can be healed and transformed has been driven by my own traumatic past, as well as my work with survivors. As a trauma survivor I know how important somatic interventions can be in taking control of one's bodily experience once again. Hypervigilance, hyperarousal, anxiety, panic attacks, and feeling overwhelmed have been my constant companions all my adult life. Gradually, I learned how body-oriented psychotherapy can moderate these symptoms and help to restore a sense of self-regulation.

Wilhelm Reich, the father of body-oriented psychotherapy, was the first to write about how the dynamics that drive abuse work within the psyche (Reich, 1970). Living in Germany when the Nazis were coming to power, he observed the dynamics of character structure inherent in the capacity for brutality and racial hatred. Many others who have written on this topic support Reich's original ideas of how splitting, projection, repression, and dissociation work within the psyche to allow one to perpetrate the utmost horror on his or her fellow human beings. Recently we have observed the extreme brutality acted out in the numerous wars in Central and South America. Currently we are witnessing the eruption of centuries-old hatreds in the cruel and ruthless destruction of human life in the former Yugoslavia. When untreated, trauma and the accompanying symptoms are passed on from generation to generation and are manifest in the acting out of perpetrators and victims.

This book evolved out of years of personal and professional work. I have taught most of the material in this book in classes or workshops in the United States, Europe, and Central America. I am deeply grateful to my students for their provocative questions and our lively discussions, which stimulated my thinking, thereby greatly enhancing the development of my ideas in this area.

MARYANNA ECKBERG

Berkeley, California
April, 1999

## Chapter One

———— ❦ ————

# SHOCK TRAUMA AND A
# SOMATIC PERSPECTIVE

### DEVELOPMENTAL TRAUMA AND SHOCK TRAUMA

Shock trauma, originally defined by Freud as a breaching of the protective stimulus barrier, can be differentiated from developmental trauma. Developmental trauma involves interruptions or distortions in normal development, which result in characterological patterns that impair healthy functioning. For instance, early deprivation caused by a mother who was unable to meet her child's emotional needs results in characterological issues related to trust. The person has difficulty being able to move out in the world and have her needs met. To compensate for underlying longing, she denies her own needs and becomes a rock, being there for others. Circumstances that shape character structure and contribute to developmental trauma may be extremely debilitating, creating serious impairment in functioning. However, there are important differences between these situations and those that involve states of shock, which result in an extreme activation of the nervous system, the flight/fight responses, reflexive reactions, and intense emotional arousal.

In shock trauma the organism is overwhelmed beyond its capacity to cope and enters into a state of shock. Its organization is profoundly altered. The entire system of perceiving, thinking, and behaving changes. There is no continuity between the past and the present. As with developmental trauma, the younger the age when the trauma occurs, the more disruption there is to the developing sense of self. Trauma can involve repeated and ongoing overwhelming events occurring during an entire childhood of abuse. For example, survivors of childhood torture are unfamiliar with anything other than a survival mode of functioning, and they must gradually learn another way of being in the world. Or trauma can involve a single incident, such as an accident, a medical procedure, or a physical assault, in persons who have lived otherwise normal lives. Political torture encompasses elements of both. Often survivors of political torture have lived normal lives that are interrupted by an ordeal which ends with their release. However, from the time of capture or arrest until the time of release the person experiences multiple incidents that are overwhelming beyond his capacity to cope. In addition, many torture survivors have experienced more than one incident of torture.

When shock trauma occurs in childhood, developmental trauma and shock trauma are interwoven. Experiences of shock trauma in the first three months of life, especially when occurring repeatedly, tend to shape a character structure based on the shock organization. For instance, the character structure identified as the *schizoid structure* or *existence structure* in body-oriented psychotherapy terminology is very similar to the *shock structure* we observe in adults who have been traumatized later in life. When shock trauma occurs after maturity, the basic character structure is more apparent, and the physical shock structure is more obvious as something almost laid on top of the character structure. It is also much easier to work with and to alter. Additionally, when shock trauma occurs after maturity, whatever developmental issues a person struggles with will be greatly exacerbated. New issues will be triggered (e.g., the right to exist, to trust others, to be autonomous; to depend on others).

The way traumatic experience manifests in the body is referred to as the shock structure. Characteristics are a marked contraction in the diaphragm, greatly restricting breathing; constriction of the tissue overall, with particularly strong tensions at the base of the skull and in the sacrum; a withdrawal of energy to the center of the body and up out of the legs and the feet; and a shrinking and bracing in the body's overall physical organization.

## HALLMARKS OF SHOCK TRAUMA

Although the psychological components of various traumatic events may differ, there are many commonalities, especially in the biological realm, among all shock trauma experiences. Traumatic shock results in a constellation of symptoms now commonly referred to as *posttraumatic stress disorder* (PTSD). Symptoms of PTSD can be categorized according to how one basically organizes oneself to relate to the world. PTSD was first defined and included in the *DSM-III* in 1980. As a formal diagnostic category, PTSD opened the door (closed long ago after the work of Freud, Janet, and Charcot) to the acknowledgment and study of the impact of overwhelming real-life events on an individual's biological, psychological, and social functioning.

At least twelve responses to shock trauma are discussed extensively in the literature:

1.  Inability to modulate arousal

2.  Intrusion of traumatic elements

3.  Somatization disorders

4. Reenactment of parts of the traumatic experience

5. Numbing and avoidance of anything related to the trauma

6. Dissociation

7. Loss of flexibility in responding to life situations

8. Disruption of attachment bonds

9. Immobility

10. Modification of one's personal identity and view of the world

11. A deep sense of shame at having let oneself down

12. The creation of a posttraumatic identity involving rigid posttraumatic defenses.[1]

## INABILITY TO MODULATE AROUSAL

One of the most common and devastating effects of shock trauma is its effect on a person's capacity to modulate autonomic arousal. Traumatized individuals continue to respond to their environment as dangerous and threatening long after the traumatic event or events. They are hypervigilant. They experience exaggerated startle responses and often have difficulty relaxing. They feel driven and restless, and they overreact to apparently minor events. Trauma survivors frequently feel overwhelmed by ordinary life events. They suffer from chronic anxiety, panic attacks, and rage attacks. The survivor's own body feels out of control and becomes a source of fear. Underlying this problem of hyperarousal are complex psychological and biological processes, which are addressed in the following sections.

One of my clients, a survivor of political torture, told me, with a puzzled look on his face, "I am afraid all of the time—afraid, like I am going to be killed. I don't understand it. Why am I always so afraid?" This man had escaped from his native country shortly after being held captive and tortured, then witnessing the execution of his wife. He had been in the United States for about nine months and had obtained political asylum. Currently he was living in a stable and very safe environment. He knows in his cognitive mind that he is now safe. This knowledge, however, is constantly overridden by another "knowing" in the more primitive parts of his brain that are still prepared to meet a life or death threat to his survival.

I have just begun working with a client who is unable to control her rage. She feels frightened and distressed, because at times she is so overcome by her anger that she cannot think rationally. She acts it out in ways that are destructive to those around her and, ultimately, self-destructive. Later she realizes that her outburst was totally irrational, and she feels guilty and dismayed by her behavior. But this does not prevent a future attack. Her cognition continues to be overridden by a reflexive fight response to a perceived threat, that is still engraved in the lower, reptilian part of her brain.

Various modes of expressing feeling overwhelmed run through the language of survivors: "Life is too much; I just can't handle it all; I feel like I am coming apart; I feel sick; everything feels out of control; I am exhausted all the time, even when I get plenty of sleep."

## INTRUSION OF TRAUMATIC ELEMENTS

By definition shock trauma cannot be integrated and digested the way normal life events are. Memories of shock trauma tend to consist of sensory impressions, somatic sensations, intense emotions, and disconnected images of what actually happened. These fragments of the traumatic experience intrude into present-day life. The intrusions may take many forms, but all involve reliving certain elements of the traumatic experience, often as vividly and intensely as the original trauma. They plague the survivor in the form of flashbacks, nightmares, traumatic imagery, panic attacks, or rage attacks. The person may experience somatic symptoms, paralysis or immobility, or behavioral reenactments. Unfortunately, replaying the trauma leads to increased, rather than decreased sensitization, as if with each replay the groove is dug deeper and leads to even more distress.

Rosa is from El Salvador. She fled from her native country seven years ago because her life was seriously threatened during the brutal civil war. She is chronically exhausted from insomnia. "I go to sleep and see blood, lots of blood and bodies all cut up." The bodies of two of her brothers were found mutilated and bearing obvious signs of torture. "I wake up and feel blood dripping on me; I try to wipe it off and then realize that it is not there."

Edith, a survivor of political torture, had incomplete escape responses burned into her nervous system, which would become activated under certain circumstances. She had been held captive in the mountains, out in the open, rather than in an enclosed room. There were many moments when she experienced the urge to run away, but at the same time knew that if she did so she would be killed. Now, even though she is living in a safe environment, she sometimes runs out of her house when something happens. The impulse to run has no direction—she just runs with no destination in mind. In psychotherapy we were working through her traumatic experiences. At times she would get up and want to leave my office in the middle of the session, flooded with an impulse to flee. I would encourage her to sense the impulses and to carefully track them by focusing on the sensations in her body. Often at the end of the session she would linger in my office, apparently not wanting to leave (suggesting that wanting to leave earlier was because of the intrusive fleeing response).

Another survivor of political torture reported that she would see images of her horrific experiences roll through her mind like a movie and would feel helpless to stop them. A survivor of childhood torture experienced symptoms of lung congestion that her doctors could not diagnose. These intrusive body memories lasted for about five weeks, until they eventually "made sense" as part of a traumatic memory involving fire and the inhalation of smoke. A client suffering from fibromyalgia discovered that the parts of her body where she suffers the most serious pain are the exact locations where she had experienced multiple severe physical traumas, some recently, and others dating back to her childhood.

## SOMATIZATION

The relationship between trauma and somatization has been known since the 1800s. Early descriptions of hysteria, relating trauma and extreme stress, form the basis of the current diagnosis of somatization disorder. A person who fails to integrate the dissociated elements of traumatic events (sensation, image, behavior, affect, meaning or knowledge) often somatically relives separated fragments of the experience.

Studies since 1980 have consistently shown a high correlation between abuse, dissociation, and somatization (van der Kolk, 1996). In one study more than 90 percent of women with somatization disorder reported histories of abuse. The total number of somatic symptoms was directly related to the DES (measure of dissociation) score (Pribor et al., 1993). Recent studies of dissociative patients indicate that somatization rarely occurs in the absence of a severe history of trauma (van der Kolk et al., 1993; Saxe et al., 1994).

Current research indicates that there is a relationship between immune system functioning and trauma. It is well known that flight/fight physiology may suppress or overactivate the immune system. Research also demonstrates that low levels of emotional expression lead to the impairment of immune system functioning and to an increase in physical illness (Spiegel, 1992; Pennebaker, 1993).

Clinical observation and research suggest there is a relationship between alexithymia and trauma (Krystal, 1988). Alexithymia is the inability to use words to identify somatic experiences physically. In normal development a child learns to interpret bodily states as emotions and as cues for action (behavior). But traumatized persons experience a progressive blocking of emotions and inhibited behavior. Researchers hypothesize that the chronic hyperarousal of traumatized persons results in a loss of their ability to differentiate the meaning of bodily feelings. Thus, trauma leads to a dedifferentiation of affects; that is, to the loss of the ability to identify and to verbalize emotions. Chronically hyperaroused, unable to put bodily experience into words, and not knowing what to do, traumatized persons are vulnerable to undifferentiated affective storms, which manifest as bodily dysfunction.

This development of alexithymia is believed to be central in the somatic symptoms typical of traumatized persons. Research by Pennebaker (1993) indicates that learning to verbalize somatic states and to reassociate them with appropriate actions decreases psychosomatic symptoms.

## REENACTMENT

It is widely observed that once an individual has been traumatized, parts of the traumatic experience will be reenacted in some way. Although not included in the diagnostic criteria for PTSD, this compulsive repetition of parts of traumatic events is seen in a broad variety of trauma survivors: combat soldiers, torture survivors, survivors of childhood abuse, accident victims, and persons who have experienced certain medical procedures. For instance, abuse survivors often find themselves again in situations where they are being victimized, or they may victimize others. Accident victims frequently find themselves involved in one accident after another. Persons who have experienced traumatic medical procedures often live with a series of somatic ailments for which there is no medical cure.

## REENACTMENT SCHEMAS

Freud observed that persons tend to repeat particular patterns of relating to the world. He called this the repetition compulsion. Schemas formed in the psyche from past experience provide the basis for this re-creation of what one has lived.

A schema may be defined as a self-perpetuating, cognitive, affective, physical, and interpersonal way of relating to the world. Schemas shape one's view of the world, which, in turn, shapes the world in a way that confirms one's working model. Information that is not consistent with the schema or model is discounted or simply not noticed: "You only live the life you see."

Reliving of normal past experience is well understood in the field of dynamic psychotherapy and psychoanalysis. When traumatic shock enters the picture, reliving the past becomes more intense, more destructive, and even more deeply in-grained. In my experience, reenactment of traumatic events seems to be less well understood. Repetitive reenactment of past traumatic events may take various forms. The survivor may play the role of either the victim or the victimizer.

## VICTIMIZATION OF OTHERS

Reenactment by a victim who becomes a perpetrator of abuse is a major cause of violence in the family and in society. Often whole societies reenact the violence, splitting into perpetrators and victims. This can be observed in various political "hot spots" around the world today, such as in Central and South America, the Middle East, and parts of Africa.

Violent criminals frequently were physically and sexually abused as children (Groth, 1979; Seghorn, Boucher, and Prentky, 1987). Studies have also found a relationship between child abuse and subsequent victimization of others (Lewis and Balla, 1976; Lewis et al., 1979). Understanding this powerful phenomenon sheds light on many behaviors that otherwise seem to make little sense.

## REVICTIMIZATION

Repeatedly living out the role of victim is another way to compulsively reenact past traumatic events. Revictimization may occur in many forms of personal interaction. Thus, rape victims are more likely to be raped again, battering relationships are repeated time and again, and assault victims are frequently assaulted again. Survivors often live through a series of events in which they are exploited in one form or another by others. In general, persons (especially women) abused as children are more likely to be abused as adults. (van der Kolk, 1989; 1996). A survivor of political torture, whom I treated, twice reenacted a captive situation involving members of her husband's family. Although she was basically "held captive," there were plenty of opportunities to escape, reminiscent of her torture experience.

## SELF-DESTRUCTIVENESS

Self-destructiveness is another form of trauma reenactment. It may include suicide attempts, cutting, burning, self-starvation, drug and alcohol abuse, and exposing oneself to dangerous situations. Studies consistently find a significant relationship between early abuse and self-harm later in life.[2] Clinicians have observed a relationship between self-mutilation and a childhood history of physical and sexual abuse or repeated surgeries (Briere, 1988; Pattison and Kahan, 1983).

## OVERWORK AND SENSATION-SEEKING

Another avenue of reenactment is addiction to action or sensation-seeking. Both allow the person to maintain a state of hyperarousal similar to that experienced during the trauma and also result in a high level of endorphin production. These types of behavioral reenactment also reactivate the emotional/cognitive program related to the trauma, that of survival-related coping mechanisms. Present-day challenges are created that require strategies of operating reminiscent of the original trauma. Thus, the person feels a sense of mastery and success that generally is lacking in ordinary life. For instance, stunt men or others who pursue risky, dangerous careers or sports are frequently reliving traumatic situations.

Trauma survivors often create crises to face. A former client of mine created a constant stream of crises in her daily life, in the drug rehabilitation programs she attended, in her psychotherapy with me, and in her psychotherapy group. This ended only when we began to treat this as a reenactment related to her severely abusive childhood.

Overwork is a common reenactment pattern. A very successful client of mine had for years kept herself overextended in her work and under constant time pressure, which gave her a sense of emergency and hyperarousal. She always felt satisfied when she could "pull it all off." At some point she realized that her coping strategies were a repeat of those that had pulled her through the original trauma (hold it all together, keep pushing, negate basic personal needs, persevere even if it seems hopeless).

## ACCIDENTS AND MEDICAL PROCEDURES

Repeated accidents and medical procedures may also be considered trauma reenactments. One client, who presented with symptoms of chronic physical pain, gradually revealed a history of eight bizarre accidents and finally disclosed a childhood history of severe physical abuse. Another client informed me that within the same year after she almost died in a serious accident, she was involved in two more accidents, which landed her in the hospital once again. Slowly, she revealed a long series of medical interventions and procedures dating back to when she was four

years old. A forty-year-old man I am currently treating presented me with a list of sixteen serious surgeries and other
medical interventions, beginning with a tonsillectomy when he
was two.

## WHAT CAUSES REENACTMENT?

Many theories attempt to explain reenactment. One is that
repetition of the familiar has survival value, because it worked
during the original trauma. Freud, who proposed the concept
of the repetition compulsion, believed that it was an attempt
to master the situation and resolve feelings of helplessness.
However, clinical experience does not support the notion that
mastery occurs. For one thing, the person is attempting to deal
with the reenacted traumatic event using an outdated model,
i.e., the schema that failed to prevent the original trauma.

The biological and neurophysiological events related to the
shock trauma provide important information about the compelling behavior of reenactment. These events include attempts
to complete the thwarted flight/fight responses; striving to discharge energy held in the nervous system; interference with the
normal functioning of the orienting responses necessary to navigate safely in the world; and addiction to one's own bodily secretions associated with states of shock.

Levine (1991, 1997) refers to the trauma vortex as a highly
charged neuro-network configuration in the nervous system.
Along with the biochemical secretions associated with trauma
(van der Kolk, 1989, 1996), it results in a powerful compulsion to
enter the trauma vortex and to reenact parts of the traumatic
event. The strength of the pull to enter the trauma vortex was
graphically demonstrated by a client who nearly died in a bicycle accident. As we were working slowly and carefully to track
the various levels of her experience of the accident, her body
would repeatedly form itself into the position it had assumed

upon impact. She would say, "It is so amazing, the pull to go here; it is so powerful—like a magnet."

Attachment theory offers explanations for interpersonal reenactments in the persistent repetition of attachment schemas originating early in life. A wide body of research on traumatic bonding indicates that when violence enters the picture, there is an increase in the intensity of the attachment bond, which cuts across species (both animals and humans experience it). In the face of danger there is an increased attachment. Explanations for this are both psychological and biological (van der Kolk, 1989). In general, attachment schemas laced with violence and danger are likely to be repeated, especially those laid down in the psyche early in life.

## AVOIDANCE AND NUMBING

Trauma survivors commonly experience a constriction in their experience of themselves and the world, resulting in a gradual detachment from ordinary life. Their withdrawal may lead to extreme isolation, which in turn may be retraumatizing, because isolation itself is usually part of the original trauma. This is especially true for survivors of childhood torture and political torture. However, I have also observed this constriction resulting in the tendency to withdraw and to isolate in survivors of nonabusive trauma such as accidents.

Survivors may avoid all stimuli that could remind them of the trauma, using drugs and alcohol to blunt their awareness, or dissociating certain experiences from their conscious awareness. Numbing of emotional and sensory experience also protects survivors from reexperiencing the painful and overwhelming emotions and physiological arousal associated with the traumatic events.

A survivor of political torture I treated had no personal friends when she began treatment, even though she had lived in this country for eight years. Her only contacts were her children, her husband (who was also highly traumatized and from whom she felt very estranged), and the people for whom she worked.

A survivor of childhood torture expressed her grief over her narrow and restricted life. After overcoming years of addiction to drugs and alcohol, which afforded her a more expansive, though blunted, life, she has remained sober. Even though she now lives a sane, organized life, she feels emotionally overwhelmed by ordinary experiences, especially those involving certain types of human interaction. She craves more in her life, yet she fears the new at the same time.

## DISSOCIATION

A major defense in shock trauma is dissociation. Dissociation is an unconscious defense mechanism and a particular way of organizing experience. It refers to "splitting off" elements of an experience from the mainstream of one's consciousness or from one's sense of self. Simply defined, dissociation means that the normal connections between thoughts, feelings, sensations, behaviors, and images are broken; things that normally go together are separated. Elements of traumatic events are isolated from each other. For instance, a person may feel the emotion associated with an event but have no experience of its content. Or one may experience somatosensory elements of an experience unconnected to the feelings and the content of the ordeal. Overwhelming events cannot be integrated into personal memory and identity. They remain separated from normal states of consciousness and from one's personal life story.

Another form of dissociation involves separated ego states, which contain the traumatic experience or which contain distinct affective states associated with traumatic events. Thus, in one ego state a person may be able to perform routine and even demanding tasks, uncontaminated by the traumatic material. In another ego state the same person may feel incapacitated by overwhelming fear, anger, or despair. Extreme dissociation of ego states results in the development of distinct identities containing differing cognitive, emotional, behavioral, and sensory experiences.

Persons with dissociated identity disorder (DID) may have various "alters" that are aware of different traumatic incidents and other alters that remain unaware of the traumatic experiences. Putnum (1989) defines alters as "highly discrete states of consciousness organized around a prevailing affect, own sense of self, including body image, with a limited repertoire of behavior and a set of state-dependent memories." Typically, these patients have suffered ongoing, intense physical, sexual, and psychological abuse from an early age. Fragmentation of parts of the traumatic experiences contributes to their having flashbacks, nightmares, psychosomatic symptoms, or reenactments. They may not remember the traumatic experiences. Thus, they cannot put the experiences into long-term, narrative memory, which would have given meaning to what they have lived through.

A third form of dissociation that occurs during traumatic events consists of distancing oneself from the actual experience by dissociating from one's bodily experience. Survivors of accidents, natural disasters, hostage situations, torture, and other ordeals frequently report out-of-body experiences—they see what is happening to them from a distance, generally from above. They feel a sense of unreality and depersonalization. They experience an altered sense of time and feel disoriented. Dissociating at the time of the trauma affords the person a defense against unbearable states of terror and helplessness. However, it is one of the most important predictors of subsequent development of PTSD (van der Kolk, 1996).

In my work with survivors of childhood torture and political torture I consistently see chronic dissociation from bodily experience. The bodies of these individuals have been assaulted and invaded, causing unbearable physical and emotional pain. They feel that their bodies are outside their control, and also that they are a continuing source of overwhelming sensation and emotion.

A client who survived ritualistic abuse from an early age would say to me, during the first two years of treatment when I referred to her body, "Don't even say that word." She meant it. Gradually and with gentle encouragement she learned to relate more positively to her bodily experience. Another survivor of childhood torture is still unable to refer to her bodily experience after years of therapy. I believe that this has contributed to the slowness of her recovery.

A male client, diagnosed as having dissociated identity disorder, tells me that his executive personality, who is mandated to navigate in the world and manage the practical part of his life, carries no feelings. Feelings are held in other streams of his consciousness—other alters.

Another client was so dissociated from her bodily experience that for about ten years she never cried. She remembered how strange it felt when she learned to cry again: "It felt like I didn't recognize the sound and this strange movement through my body."

When a person goes into the "black hole of trauma" and experiences intense emotional states related to the traumatic event, these states become dissociated from other elements of the traumatic event and from the reality of present experience. This means that the survivor does not realize that his or her experience comes from the past. Because of what is called mistaken source monitoring, the person attributes the emotions to something in the present. In addition, a person who enters the "black hole" dissociates from the external world. This makes it very difficult for the therapist to make the contact necessary to help the survivor realize that he or she is reliving a past event.

As another client was working through the depths of her traumatic past, her neck became frozen in a peculiar way. No hands-on work helped to relieve the discomfort. ( She tried chiropractic, cranial sacral work, massage, *jin shin jyutsu*). This was a dissociated body memory, only relieved by body-oriented emotional work on the traumatic material. By reassociating the fragmented bodily experience with the other essential pieces of the traumatic event, she finally achieved release and relief.

## Loss of Flexibility in Responding to Life Situations

Shock trauma results in a profound alteration in a person's way of perceiving, thinking about, and relating to the self and the world. Shock trauma is organized in the primitive parts of the brain—a major reason why trauma-related behavior is so difficult to change. Stimuli related to traumatic events trigger the primitive, reflexive flight/fight responses. At such times it is difficult, if not impossible, to draw on information stored in the cerebral cortex, which would let one consider options before taking action. Thus, traumatized persons have difficulty sorting out the relevant stimuli in a situation. Their capacity to experience what Freud called "thought as experimental action," is greatly impaired. They respond reflexively, as though the current situation contains the same danger as past traumatic experiences.

A survivor of political torture had been captured by the military and tortured for months. He reported that whenever he saw a man in uniform, such as a policeman, he felt terrified and compelled to run or hide. He knew that this was not rational behavior in his present life, but his emotional arousal and his behavior were reflexive and impulsive, overriding his cognitive process.

A client who returned from working in a foreign country gave an example of the inability to entertain alternatives. Making a side trip between teaching engagements, she had carefully checked train schedules to ensure that she would return in time for her next workshop. Upon her arrival at the train station, she inquired at the information desk about the location of her train. The woman in the booth told her that there was no train to her destination at that time. My client spoke the language fluently and knew that she had not misunderstood the words. She immediately flew into a state of hyperarousal. Her mind clouded over. She had the impulse to jump into a taxi to take her to her destination, which would have been extremely expensive. However, she had learned in her psychotherapy about the importance of "buying time," or taking time out to settle herself. She did this by going and staring at the board that displayed arrival and departure times of various trains.

For a moment, she began to think that it was Thursday instead of Sunday, because the board stated that on weekdays trains to her destination left at this time. But, as she stood there, grounding herself in the reality of the present, she saw that the board clearly showed that a train was leaving for her destination at this time. Only then did she notice that there was another woman at the information desk. She went to ask her for the same information, and was told that her train was right outside.

The point is that had she not gone into a trauma reaction, she would have exercised some flexibility in responding to this situation. Instead of just entering into a state of hyperarousal, concluding that she must have made a mistake and that she needed to find a survival course of action, she probably would have remembered how carefully she had checked the train schedules. She might have confronted the woman who gave her the wrong information. She might have noticed immediately that there was another woman at the information window and asked her if the information she had been given was correct.

## Disruption of Attachment Bonds

A person's general manner of relating to others is deeply affected by incidents of abuse. He withdraws from interpersonal interaction and determines to depend only on himself. He wants to avoid the intimacy of trusting another person. In addition, depending on the person's age and the defensive system he has constructed, abuse results in specific interpersonal schemas of relating that are frequently retraumatizing. Or the person may perpetuate the abuse on others.

Recent research in the biology of attachment suggests even deeper effects, which are found in all forms of trauma, including those that do not include abuse. Distress, which produces high cortisol levels and a high heart rate, is mediated by the external environment. If a person under stress is able to make contact with another caring human being, her body begins to produce natural opioids, oxytocin, and prolactin, which have a calming effect on the nervous system. A distressed person who cannot get relief from a bonding experience must do something internally, like dissociate (cortisol levels drop and opioid levels rise). In the posttraumatic period, survivors also use dissociation, reenactment, or drugs to change their biochemistry in an attempt to find relief not available to them through human contact.

Clinical observation indicates that as distress goes up, attachment breaks down. Adrenaline, norepinephrine, epinephrine increase as self-survival becomes an imperative. The secretion of prolactin, oxytocin, and the opioids is suppressed. Obviously, abuse carries much more severe implications for how a survivor will relate to others. However, research suggests that there is also a biological basis for the attachment system to shut down when the person faces any form of serious threat to survival (Henry, 1996).

A survivor of childhood torture once told me that the best she has ever felt in her life was when each of her three children were born. It was clear that these good feelings included the pregnancies and the nursing period following the births. Another client, whose attachment system had been shut down for years, found that her capacity to relate to others opened up again during the period when she gave birth to her two children. She too reported that this was the best she can ever remember feeling.

I once worked with a young man whose life had been shattered by the "disappearance"[3] of his brother and then by being held captive and tortured. Nine months before he began his work with me, he had fled for his life from his native country. It was clear to me that his character was not shy or withdrawn. Nevertheless, he initially found it difficult to be with me during the sessions. He continued to come only because he felt so desperate. He told me that he sometimes did not talk to anyone for weeks at a time, even though he went to work daily and lived with a young couple who spoke his native language. Gradually he opened up and formed a bond with me. After this he began to let a few other people into his life.

## IMMOBILITY

I believe that immobility or freezing, as part of the flight/fight response, is one of the posttraumatic symptoms least understood by clients and therapists alike. It is simply not knowing what to do and being unable to act in a situation that, realistically, is not particularly threatening. A person may find herself unable to do even a simple task. Sometimes there is a chronic problem of not being able to follow through with activities, even those that the person truly wants to do. Sometimes an underlying unresolved state of immobility is the cause of a person being unable to move forward in his life. Often, when working with traumatic material, a client will enter a very still, yet internally activated state. He or she may report feeling heavy or paralyzed and unable to move. With guidance and support from the therapist, this can be an important opportunity for reorganization on a neurophysiological level. However, when this state is not understood, entering it during sessions or between sessions can be a source of puzzlement and even alarm.

One survivor of political torture habitually entered into a state of immobility that she called "feeling lazy." She would feel as though all the energy had drained from her body, and that she could hardly move her arms or legs. Before she began treatment with me, she would often remain on her bed for long periods of time, unable to mobilize herself to get up.

The major complaint of one survivor of ritualistic childhood abuse is that she finds it difficult and at times impossible to follow through with activities, this is especially things that she really wants to do. In our work together it became clear that she has movement up to a point. Then she becomes triggered by her movement and goes into a freezing state, making it impossible to go further. In addition, she felt unable to move forward with her life in general, i.e., to go back to school or to change jobs.

A young man traumatized by series of surgeries that took place after birth and continued during the first year of his life would often sit for hours staring into space. He would be unable even to do the necessary activities to keep his home organized, because he would lose his direction and find himself immobilized. He felt stuck in his life in general. Previously he had been diagnosed with *attention deficit disorder* (ADD), and ritalin had been prescribed, but he said that it did not help him with this problem. In his interpersonal relationships he experienced outbursts of rage alternating with extreme passivity.

During therapy, while working with his early medical trauma, he frequently entered states of immobility. He felt that he was strapped down and unable to move. It became clear that the immobility was related both to an inherent part of his shock trauma and to his actual experience of having been immobilized during and after his childhood surgeries. We gradually uncoupled the terror and rage associated with this state and began to mobilize his frozen defensive and orienting responses. As we worked through this part of his trauma, he began to experience movement in his life in general and an increase in his capacity to initiate and to follow through with activities. He stopped having explosions of rage, salvaging an otherwise healthy relationship with a young woman whom he later married.

A client I had seen for only a month reported an incident that occurred during the week prior to her session. One day she was home alone in her apartment. Someone came to the door and pounded on it. Although the person obviously had the wrong apartment, she froze and sat on her bed immobilized for over an hour. All the time that she was sitting there she kept telling herself how ridiculous it was, yet she could not move. As her therapy unfolded I learned about the violent and explosive home situation in which she had lived as a young child.

## MODIFICATION OF PERSONAL IDENTITY AND WORLD VIEW

Experiencing a threat to one's life in any form, whether from a natural disaster or abuse, greatly affects one's perception of oneself and one's view of the world. When the circumstances involve abuse by fellow human beings, the consequences are devastating. One's view of the world and oneself must somehow incorporate the cruelty and the violence.

Although a person's age at the time of the trauma, previous life events, and even current life events will influence how traumatic experiences are interpreted, the idea that the world is a safe place is seriously challenged. The notion that fellow humans are basically good and just is impossible to accept. One feels helpless, humiliated, and out of control. It is difficult to count on anyone, especially oneself.

Survivors frequently lose any passion for life or even willingness to live. So often I hear from my clients who are victims of violence, "I just don't want to be here; I don't want to be alive." Such feelings should not be confused with feeling actively suicidal; they do not include an intention or a plan to take one's own life. On the contrary, typically I find this attitude fused with the intention to live one's life with as much dignity as possible.

## SHAME

Shame accompanies all experiences of shock trauma. It is the sense that one has let oneself down, that one was not able to meet the challenge. Survivors of abuse, especially torture, live with intense and very complex feelings of shame. Being unable to integrate these intense feelings often leads to further victimization or to victimizing others.

Holocaust survivor, Primo Levi, refers to the meaning of the Greek word *adios* as shame when the natural order is violated: "The shame which the just man experiences when confronted by a crime committed by another, and he feels remorse because of its existence, because of its having been irrevocably introduced into the world of living things and because his will has proven nonexistent or feeble and was incapable of putting up a good defense (Levi, 1988 ).

## FORMATION OF A POSTTRAUMATIC IDENTITY

A serious threat to survival may, over time, lead to organizing one's life and identity around a survival mode of functioning. A survivor may become a shy, withdrawn, and fearful person, who leads a constricted and isolated life. Or, the experience oneself of being highly activated, flooded, overwhelmed, and constantly overextended may become a survivor's identity.

The formation of a posttraumatic identity depends on the age of traumatization, the pretraumatic personality, and circumstances such as acceptance and support from others and availability of professional help. A posttraumatic identity is very resistant to change, given that the defensive structure was laid down in life and death situations. Surrendering the new identity may result in a feeling of falling apart. The survivor may again feel the terror associated with the original threat and the fear that he or she is going to die. He or she may even want to die, and may feel unbearably helpless. These feelings typically surface over time when a reorganization of identity is occurring. However, for healing to occur the person must gradually let go of this survival identity.

A survivor of childhood torture is feeling better than she can ever remember. She is finally managing to organize a life that is satisfying and secure. At the same time that she is recognizing this achievement, she expresses fear that she will sabotage her success. Can she tolerate feeling good and feeling good about herself? Before the next session I received a phone call. She is feeling despair, frustration, some of her old feelings of paranoia related to human interaction, and anger. Her whole perception of the world and herself has reverted to the sense of herself that she is in the process of reorganizing.

A client's posttraumatic identity is predicated on "holding it all together." Thus, she organized her life so that she was overextended and overwhelmed, proving again and again to herself how well she could hold it all together. When she was finally able to begin reorganizing this way of being, she experienced overwhelming grief and constant terror that her life would fall apart. She felt a sense of futility that threatened to paralyze her current life as it had shattered and paralyzed her life during the original trauma. Experiencing this was so painful and frightening that she clearly understood why her old way of being had been so resistant to change.

A man who suffered abuse by his mother and other family members in addition to life in a concentration camp has "fought to survive" all his life. He is convinced there is no other way to live. Relenting even a little on this firm stance, entertaining the possibility that perhaps he doesn't have to struggle always to survive, generates extreme anxiety and agitation. He desperately wants to perceive himself and the world differently, to be able to relax and enjoy the simple pleasures. However, he finds himself pulled again and again into his old position of fighting with life.

In my experience, clients who are diagnosed with dissociated identity disorder invariably react negatively to the idea of—or even the word—integration. Dissociatig parts of themselves was their survival strategy. Initially it is impossible for them to imagine another way of being. I never use the word with them nor work directly to integrate their parts. However, at some point in the therapy, they just find themselves coming together. When I point out that they appear to be doing that terrible thing called integration, they generally feel surprised and amused at themselves.

## LIFE ENERGY AND NEGATIVE EMOTIONS

When the life energy (arousal or activation) is thwarted in an attempt at protection, a significant part of the undischarged energy becomes organized into negative emotions, such as rage, terror, fear, hatred, and shame. These negative emotions become associated with the life energy itself. For instance, feeling excited about something positive is felt as anxiety or even panic. Feeling expansive becomes a sense of danger and catastrophic thinking. This is a form of *overcoupling*, i.e., two or more experiences become tightly associated (Levine, 1997).

## NEUROPHYSIOLOGICAL UNDERPINNINGS OF SHOCK TRAUMA

As a clinician with thirty years of experience, I understood years ago that healing involves the reorganization of one's experience on all levels: cognitive, emotional, physical, and energetic. My twenty-two years of experience in the area of somatic psychotherapy have taught me the importance of making interventions on a body level, as well as the cognitive and emotional levels to facilitate this. However, I am indebted to my colleague, Peter Levine, for filling in some important missing pieces for me in the treatment of shock trauma (Levine, 1991, 1997). His understanding of traumatic shock includes both clinical work and observation of the animal world and combines aspects of ethology, catastrophe theory, somatic therapies, and neurophysiological systems.

To understand the neurophysiological underpinnings of shock trauma, it is helpful to visit, for a moment, the animal world. When an animal in the wild senses danger, a series of instinctive and reflexive responses are set into motion, mediated by its autonomic nervous system. Initially, the animal goes into a state of arrest—all movement ceases. Its orienting responses are activated, and the animal scans the environment for more information. If no threat is found, the animal returns to a state of equilibrium (homeostasis) and goes on its way.

A threat, however, triggers the animal's defensive patterns of response registered in the primitive parts of the brain, mobilizing the flight/fight response. Chemicals pour into its system, its heart rate goes way up, and blood flow to the skin and other organs decreases. Pupils dilate. Muscles contract and prepare for action. The energetic charge in its body is extremely high as the animal prepares to meet a life-threatening event. This is a nonconscious process, which in humans overrides the functioning of the cerebral cortex, that part of the brain that integrates and processes information. Depending on the circumstances, the animal will move toward the threat, preparing to fight, or will flee. If escape is impossible and the animal does not have the defensive resources to fight, frenzied, nonfocused activity follows, involving feelings of terror and rage.

Finally, the animal enters a state of shock, which involves freezing, and collapse into tonic immobility. Immobility is a mechanism an organism uses to shut itself down when escape is impossible. This last-ditch stand involves an analgesic response and dissociation. Internally, the animal is physiologically highly activated; externally, there is no movement. Sympathetic and parasympathetic systems are activated simultaneously. This is somewhat like pressing the brake and accelerator in a car at the same time, resulting in concurrent hyperarousal and inhibition. In nature, the tonic immobility and the accompanying analgesia serve an adaptive function. As Levine (1991) states, "An immobile (prey) animal is . . . less likely to be detected by a predator; and if detected, it is less likely to be attacked. Further, if attacked, it is less likely to be killed and eaten, increasing its chances of escape and reproduction."

However, the flight/fight and immobility response states are adaptive only when appropriate to the situation, and only if the chain of responses is allowed to move through to completion. When flight/fight responses are appropriate, immobility is not. An important survival strategy in particular situations, immobility is maladaptive in others. Immobility may become chronic; that is, a preferred response pattern to activating stimuli in general. This means that when a survivor becomes activated physiologically, he or she bypasses the flight/fight responses altogether and goes directly into a state of immobility.

At this point in an emergency situation, the animal is either killed, or else its nervous system completes the emergency responses and returns to homeostasis. In humans this is frequently not the case. When faced with a life-threatening situation, the person is often prevented, for various reasons, from completing the chain of response states. Thus, orienting and defensive responses thwarted at the time of the trauma remain activated in the person's nervous system, unable to resolve. Fragments of the experience dissociated at the time of the trauma are unable to reassociate. In addition, images, sensations, motor patterns, and emotions related to the experience may become tightly connected, forming an uninterrupted pathway of experience called *overcoupling*.

In summary, if a person faced with an overwhelming threat is unable to flee or to fight and becomes immobilized, then he or she is likely to suffer the debilitating symptoms referred to as posttraumatic stress disorder, such as chronic hypervigilance, chronic hyperarousal, dissociation, medically untreatable psychosomatic symptoms, intrusive images, panic attacks, rage attacks, disorientation, and the inability to process cognitively when highly activated.[4]

In essence, shock trauma becomes encoded in the primitive parts of the brain. The language of the primitive part of the brain is sensation. The most direct and effective approach in work with sensation is a body-oriented psychotherapy, discussed later in this chapter.

## THE PSYCHOBIOLOGY OF TRAUMATIC SHOCK

There is a large body of research focusing on the effects of trauma on the human brain and the functioning of basic biological functions. Much of this cutting-edge research has been done by Bessell van der Kolk, who has published several excellent summaries of his own work and that of others (van der Kolk, 1987, 1989, 1996).

The human brain consists of three interdependent systems: (1) the neocortex, responsible for cognitively processing information; (2) the limbic system, important in regulating between internal experience and the external world; and (3) the brainstem and hypothalamus, which regulate internal homeostasis. Recent research shows that shock trauma affects all three of these levels, but that the undesirable results of trauma come from the altered biological functioning of the more primitive parts of the brain: the limbic system, the brainstem, and the hypothalamus. The functioning of the cerebral cortex is profoundly affected by—and, frequently overridden by—this encoding of trauma in the lower parts of the brain.

Arousal in response to perceived danger is mediated by the catecholamines: epinephrine, norepinephrine (adrenaline), and dopamine. Dissociation is mediated by the endogenous opioids (endorphins). Other stress-related hormones involved in responses to extreme stress are serotonin, cortisol, vasopressin, and oxytocin. A person's sense of well-being and capacity to respond appropriately to stimuli; to modulate arousal when activated by incoming stimuli; to relate to and bond to others, to relax, and to process cognitively are greatly affected by the balance of these neurohormones in the body. Traumatic shock alters this balance. It results in the nervous system always being "off center" and the person never being able to find refuge behind a protective stimulus barrier.

In traumatic shock the nervous system, which generally amplifies to receive stimuli and then diminishes the effect, continues to amplify. Excitation continues to increase, resulting in chronic hypervigilance and hyperarousal. In addition the nervous system becomes sensitized to stimuli, so that less and less of a stimulus is needed to elicit an ever-increasing, more widespread response. Increased levels of endogenous opioids (endorphins) under stress results in dissociation. There is also evidence (van der Kolk, 1989) that addiction to the endogenous opioids, and perhaps other hormones as well, plays an important role in trauma reenactment. In other words, the person is drawn to expose himself to highly stressful, self-destructive, and retraumatizing experiences, that encourage the release of more endorphins, serotonin, cortisol, vasopressin, and oxytocin.

Some recent and fascinating research suggests that the breakdown of the attachment system observed as a result of shock trauma also seems to have a biological component (Henry, 1996). Survivors of traumatically stressful events are often described as or describe themselves as being isolated, feeling detached from others and from life itself, finding it difficult to trust and relate to others. I have even observed this in clients who are not survivors of abuse, but who have survived traumatic events such as accidents. Thus, clinical observations, along with empirical studies, suggest that as the urgency of self-survival goes up, attachment behavior breaks down.

A summary of the very complex empirical work suggests that self and species preservation have separate hemispheric laterality and separate hormonal paths. Hormones such as prolactin, oxytocin, and the opioids increase with bonding and physical intimacy. Maternal behavior is mediated by the opioid system; that is, opioid secretion increases with contact. Mother primates who were given morphine lost interest in their infants (Soumi, 1996). These attachment related hormones appear to be associated with the functioning of the right side of the brain, which is suppressed during extreme stress. External threat elicits the flight/fight response (epinephrine, norepinephrine), leading to depression of right hemispheric functioning and the production of attachment-related hormones, such as oxytocin, prolactin, and the opioids (Henry, 1996).

## TRAUMA AND MEMORY

*I have been waiting for some vital shock to take place, some deep, extended nightmare to explode suddenly in the middle of the night, allowing me to relive it all—something that will take me back to the original scene, purify me, and then restore me to this place where I am now writing. But nothing has happened, and I find this calm terrifying.*[5]

The recognition that memory of traumatic events is laid down in the mind differently than memory of normal events dates back to the very foundation of psychoanalysis, psychology, and psychiatry. Janet, Charcot, Breuer, and Freud all observed that memories of frightening events do not appear to be integrated, assimilated, and retrieved in the same manner as memories for ordinary, everyday events. These early clinicians (Janet, in particular) developed complex ideas about how traumatic memory is stored in the brain and the impact of this, in turn, on experience and behavior. Janet observed that traumatic memory manifests as sensation, affect, behavior, or images; that is, as somatosensory information. At the time of the trauma these perceptual experiences are stored in the body (van der Kolk and van der Hart, 1989). This important early work was later pushed aside by the developmental directions that psychoanalysis and psychiatry took.

Contemporary research has confirmed the work of these early

pioneers and has broadened and deepened our understanding of memory in general, and of how traumatic memory differs in qualitatively important ways. "Traumatic memory consists of emotional and sensory states with little verbal representation. The hippocampal-based memory categorization system fails, leaving memory to be stored as affective and perceptual states" (van der Kolk and Fisler, 1995, p. 513). Thus, images, sensations, emotions, and behavior occurring at the time of the trauma are preserved in the body dissociated from each other and from the knowledge of what happened.

Clinicians have long recognized that there are two rudimentary forms of memory: conscious and unconscious. Most memory functioning occurs outside of conscious awareness. Memory is a neural-network configuration related to processing incoming stimulation, integrating it with existing mental schemas, and retrieving it. Retrieval involves a neural activation profile similar to that at the time of encoding.

Declarative memory (also called reflective memory) is conscious and refers to that which can be stated, like facts and events. It involves symbolic language and narrative skills. Perceptual memory (also called procedural memory) is unconscious and refers to memories of sensations, behavioral skills, emotional responses, and reflexive actions. Emotional memory exists in both these forms. One has feelings both about what one knows and what one sees and smells (Squire, 1994).

Another way of categorizing memory, which is probably most relevant to traumatic memory and body-oriented work, is as explicit or implicit memory. This distinction involves the sequencing of how incoming information is processed and assimilated by existing mental schemas. Focal attention is crucial at each step in the process of sorting, categorizing, and associating incoming material with already existing memory. During traumatic events, focalized attention is seriously disrupted.

Explicit memory includes declarative memory. It is conscious and automatically integrated; it can be stated, reflected upon, retrieved, and put into narrative form. Implicit memory, on the other hand, is nonconscious and involves somatosensory experience. It is similar to what is referred to as perceptual memory (Siegel, 1993). Since the time of Janet, clinical observation has emphasized that traumatic experiences are imprinted on a perceptual, nonverbal level. The trauma is remembered as fragments of sensory experience, such as smells, sounds, body sensations, behavioral enactments, or intense feelings. The perceptions are usually reported as exact representations of parts of the original experience, as though the person were experiencing it in present time. However, there is no narrative for the event that explains the fragmentary somatosensory experience. The story of what happened must be constructed from these memory fragments. On the other hand the encoding of ordinary events, resulting in explicit memory is automatically integrated and organized into a narrative.

The relationship between implicit and explicit memory is extremely important in understanding traumatic memory, trauma resolution, and the importance of a body-oriented approach in the treatment process. Research and clinical observation supports the idea that traumatic experience is encoded in such a way that it still lives inside the person as though it were happening in the present. It is remembered as a reexperiencing of the event, rather than as a story placed in time, typical of narrative memory. Thus, traumatized persons are unable to acknowledge what really happened to them, to integrate it, and to go on with their lives (Schacter, 1987).

A client's life was shattered by a traumatic event. Relatively benign, unexpected events trigger the feeling that she is fragmenting, and that her life is falling apart. A survivor of political torture, who had been held by soldiers in the mountains, fled blindly from numerous situations, before she acknowledged and integrated the idea that the fleeing impulse related to her having been held captive. Years after surviving a serious accident, a client finds herself in a work situation in which she feels relatively powerless. The situation repeatedly triggers the feeling of extreme helplessness she felt during and after her traumatic accident.

Current research has provided important information to explain what happens neurophysiologically during traumatic events.[6] A different encoding process takes place. In a primitive part of the brain, the limbic system, there are three areas important in the processing of frightening and emotionally charged experiences. The first is the locus ceruleus, which functions as the alarm bell, triggering the secretion of norepinephrine, mobilizing the organism to mobilize to meet an emergency. The second structure is the amygdala, which evaluates the relevance of incoming stimuli. It assigns significance to sensory input, evaluating the emotional meaning of the incoming information, and then directs this to the third area, the hippocampus and related structures.

The hippocampus plays an important role in categorizing new information and integrating it with existing mental schemas. For explicit, declarative, or narrative memory to exist, incoming stimuli must be processed by the hippocampus, which takes weeks to months. When the amygdala is highly stimulated, it interferes with proper functioning of the hippocampus. The intense stimulation of the amygdala will prevent a traumatic experience from being explicitly remembered.

In addition, explicit memory requires focal attention on incoming stimuli, resulting in reflection on the perceptual content. During traumatic events, the flight/fight response and accompanying hormonal stimulation produce high states of arousal, making focal attention impossible. Thus, the incoming stimuli cannot be categorized, digested, and stored as long-term memory. The information is remembered through a different system outside of cortical and hippocampal control.

The experience is registered as implicit memory. It consists of perceptual, rather than reflective content. It is then remembered (relived) as body sensations, emotions, images, and motoric behavior. This high perceptual content, which is vividly experienced with little capacity for reflection, results in mistaken source monitoring. One tends to misinterpret external experience because of internal perceptual cues which are related to past, not present experience. Current experience is distorted and perceived as a potential threat.

The way an individual processes implicit memory into explicit, declarative memory is central to his or her treatment for PTSD. The somatosensory nature of traumatic memory implies the usefulness of a somatic psychological orientation, that is, a treatment approach that is anchored in sensory experience.

The concepts of repression and dissociation are frequently used interchangeably to explain unconscious traumatic memory. However, the two processes are quite different. In the sequence of memory processing (perceive, register, store, retrieve), repression is related to the storage and retrieval components. Dissociation is associated with the initial phases of perceiving and registering incoming stimuli. In addition, repression involves a vertical layering in the mind; repressed material is pushed downward into the unconscious. Dissociation, on the other hand, reflects a horizontal separation. Parts of an experience are held in various streams of consciousness. The "not remembering" of an event occurs when the state of consciousness in which it is contained is eclipsed by other states of consciousness.

In shock trauma, parts of the traumatic experience fragment and generally are not reassociated, resulting in amnesic barriers between various elements. Thus, sensations related to a traumatic event may be experienced unrelated to images of what happened. Behavioral reenactments may occur, with no understanding of their meaningful connection to the original experience. One may be swept by emotions of terror, rage, helplessness, and despair. Images of the traumatic event may run through one's mind like a movie, disconnected from affect or sensation. These dissociated and undigested fragments of traumatic experience produce what are commonly referred to as flashbacks, psychosomatic symptoms, reenactments, and nightmares. Parts of the trauma are relived instead of being remembered or recalled in the sense of being reflected upon, as is the case in normal memory.

Dissociated memory is retrieved and becomes conscious when the person is in a state of mind similar to the one in which the encoding took place. This is called *state-dependent memory*: If the state of consciousness during recall is similar to the state of consciousness during the original experience, the memory is recalled. Thus, just feeling excited (in a high state of arousal) may lead to remembering or reliving parts of the traumatic experience. Trauma survivors may feel and act as though they are being traumatized once again. Remembering or reliving the trauma, in turn, leads to hyperarousal. This vicious circle includes a tendency to distort current external experience as sources of danger. This is why dissociative memory results in bouts of emotional flooding, flashbacks, panic attacks, and nightmares.

Intrusive sensations and affective states related to the trauma are not extinguished by processing the experiences on a linguistic level and constructing a narrative of the event (van der Kolk, 1996). Contrary to a basic assumption in many forms of treatment, these elements of the traumatic experience continue to intrude into present-day living even after a survivor can "tell the whole story."

## BODY-ORIENTED PSYCHOTHERAPY

Body-oriented psychotherapy is a branch of psychotherapy based on a distinct and explicit theory of mind-body functioning and on the relationship between the various levels of experience—cognitive, emotional, physical, and energetic. It is a way of understanding personality, or character structure, through one's bodily experiences and energetic processes. This is an integrative and holistic orientation, making no distinction between the mind and the body. Recent research (Paired) supports the notion that the mind resides throughout the body, and that every cell in the body stores information or "thinks" and communicates with other cells.

Body-oriented or somatic psychotherapy "involves a developmental model; a theory of personality; hypotheses as to the origins of disturbances and alterations, as well as a rich variety of diagnostic and therapeutic techniques used within the framework of the therapeutic relationship" (European Association for Body-Oriented Psychotherapy, 1995). It has a long tradition, dating back to the work of Wilhelm Reich, M.D., psychoanalyst and student of Sigmund Freud (Reich, 1961a, 1961b). Alexander Lowen (1958, 1965, 1972, 1978) and John Pierrakos (1973, 1987), both psychiatrists, built on Reich's groundbreaking foundation and expanded this knowledge. A somatic psychotherapy called bioenergetics grew out of this effort and is the most well known of the body-oriented approaches.

Stanley Keleman (Keleman, 1975, 1979, 1985); Lisbeth Marcher in Denmark (McNaughten, 1996); and others have also added to the knowledge of the body-oriented psychotherapeutic approach. This orientation emphasizes that one's history is structured in one's body; that all one has lived through is embodied. How a person meets, deals with, and integrates developmental challenges forms the personality or character structure and is structured in the body. As in all forms of psychotherapeutic theory and practice, unresolved issues manifest as problems. In working therapeutically with these problems, the therapist observes how a client's body is organized, how the client is responding somatically, and how the client reports his or her bodily experience. These observations provide a great deal of additional information, which guides the therapist in making interventions on a body level as well as a verbal level.

# Chapter Two

———— ⚬❀⚬ ————

# THE CLINICAL PROCESS:
# A SOMATIC ORIENTATION

*Since then, at an uncertain hour,*
*That agony returns,*
*And till my ghastly tale is told*
*This heart within me burns*

COLERIDGE,
*THE RIME OF THE ANCIENT MARINER*

Survivors of shock trauma experience their bodies as being out of control. In fact, their neurophysiology and biology are out of control in that the normal capacity to modulate arousal has been seriously affected. It is apparent that traumatic memory consists primarily of sensation, perceptual experience, behavioral responses, and affective states, with little verbal representation; that is, traumatic memory is somatosensory experience. Traumatic memory is primarily dissociated memory. It is retrieved as sensory experience, somatic experience, intense emotion, perceptual impressions, images or behavior, not as verbally intact memory.

The symptoms suffered by survivors of shock trauma (PTSD) involve principally the lower, more primitive parts of the brain. Those who understand the somatic psychotherapeutic approach know that sensory information is as important as cognitive and emotional knowledge. Awareness of body sensation is enormously helpful when working with developmental issues, but is even more important when working with shock trauma. Body sensation is a direct doorway to the unconscious mind. Cognitive restructuring is, of course, important, but the healing process must include bodily experience.

Somatic interventions, therefore, provide information as to how a traumatic experience is physiologically patterned and help to access biological resources to undo these patterns. By working on a body level with the somatosensory experience of the survivor, one can communicate directly with the primitive parts of the brain and the unconscious mind, addressing the symptoms of PTSD and facilitating the reorganization of traumatic material.

Professionals in the field of trauma generally agree that healing requires remembering and, in some way, processing the traumatic material (van der Kolk, 1996). What remains unclear is just how to do this. Talking about a shock experience is likely to leave out important elements. Parts of the experience may be dissociated and thus be inaccessible. Verbal therapies may achieve a cognitive reorganization but leave the physiological, motoric, and emotional underpinnings untouched.

On the other hand, therapeutic approaches that subscribe to cathartic release risk retraumatizing the patient. Reliving a traumatic event, partially or fully, not only does not heal, but very likely just digs even more deeply the grooves of the neuro-network configuration that organizes traumatic symptomatology.

Uncontrolled abreactive states may emerge in verbal therapies when therapists are not trained to deal with the terror, rage, and immobility. Somatic psychotherapists, unfamiliar with shock trauma, are likely to uncover shock material, because somatic interventions are particularly effective in this regard. Shock experiences are highly charged. When they are uncovered, the intensity of the physiological responses and emotions involved may leave a client feeling, once again, totally helpless and out of control. Cathartic work that floods the client with emotional and physiological responses related to the trauma results in the therapeutic situation feeling unsafe and undermines trust in the therapist. The hydraulic discharge model of working with trauma—the idea that the traumatic experience can be bled out—is out of date.

There are three phases of treatment in which a body-based approach is particularly important. The first is the initial stage of education, containment, and stabilization. The second phase of treatment in which a somatic orientation seems crucial is in renegotiating the traumatic material in order to integrate it into the survivor's sense of self and into a coherent personal narrative. In the third phase, a body-oriented approach can help traumatized clients reestablish their capacity for pleasure and positive experiences.

## PHASE ONE:
## EDUCATION, CONTAINMENT, AND STABILIZATION

The therapeutic relationship is the foundation of all psychotherapeutic approaches. In the treatment of shock trauma the healing process must be embedded in the client's secure attachment to the therapist, who is trusted to help the survivor modulate and regulate emotional arousal when renegotiating traumatic memories. The therapist's office will not feel safe if a client finds herself reliving past trauma, flooding with intense emotion, and leaving the session feeling disorganized, fearful, and vulnerable. Indispensable in the treatment process is the strong empathic presence of the therapist and his or her capacity to contain the horror and suffering communicated by the survivor. The therapist must be able to understand the survivor's experience and to convey this to him, and must be able to maintain clear boundaries. Once conditions for creating a safe environment have been met, the skill of the therapist in helping the survivor renegotiate and integrate traumatic material also becomes important.

Working somatically, I am able to see and monitor the client's somatic responsiveness, while at the same time remaining connected to my own bodily experience. Demonstrating to survivors that I am able to address their distressing symptoms with tangible interventions often brings them a sense of relief and supports the belief that my office is a safe place to bring their suffering. Attention to the body takes the pressure off, so the client doesn't feel he must talk about what happened. I know that by working on a body level the whole story will eventually emerge at the client's own pace. Conveying this to the client encourages building trust.

I bring clients to an awareness of how they are organized physically, what they do on a body level when they dissociate or begin to become hyperaroused. This makes it easier for them to understand their symptoms and experience how they are related to the flight/fight sequence of events: preparation for emergency, impulses to flee or to fight, disorganized frenzy, immobility and dissociation.

A certain survivor of political torture suffers from insomnia and nightmares, among other common symptoms of PTSD. She always feels fatigued, but is unable to rest because of her chronic state of hypervigilance and hyperarousal. Trust and rapport was established relatively easily. She was quite willing to work somatically and always left the sessions feeling much less anxious, more present in herself, and even relaxed and "tired." After a few sessions, each time she came she reported feeling tired on the way to the session, and felt her fatigue even more in the waiting room. She seemed bewildered by this. She described the tired feeling as positive, not negative; the sense of letting down instead of holding up and together. What she meant became clearer when she began to talk about how peaceful it is in my office, how safe it feels. That feeling of safety in my office provides the holding environment in which she can do her work. I believe the somatic work facilitated this. It also allowed her to contact places of feeling safe in herself, which she takes with her into the world.

Educating survivors about their symptoms is an important first step in treatment. Survivors of extreme experiences, whether violent abuse, such as torture, or an accident, frequently feel very confused about what they are experiencing. Often they fear that they are going crazy because of the in-tensity of their emotions and their physiological arousal. Feeling so out of control in itself is frightening. Providing a cognitive frame in which survivors can hold their extraordinary experiences helps them to feel less abnormal and to understand that their current distress is related to these past traumatic events.

Each survivor is different and must be met in a way that he or she can understand. I once had to explain in Spanish to an Indian from Guatemala the meaning of his distressing symptoms. He was twenty years old, but he had not learned to speak Spanish (he had spoken only his Indian dialect) until he was eighteen. Among his other symptoms of PTSD, he remembered nothing of his life from age twelve to eighteen. His dissociation in the present was quite apparent. I had to create unusual ways to help him understand his symptoms. His responsiveness suggested that he understood me. Within three sessions he was markedly less dissociative.

In general, what I convey to each person is similar. I explain that he or she has lived one or a series of extreme experiences, outside the normal range of human experience; that a person is unable to cope with such experiences the way one can cope with normal experiences. Therefore, the person (or animal; I often talk about the experiences of animals, as this seems to normalize it even more) must find different ways to survive. These ways of surviving are very important at the time, but if they persist, they become the distressing symptoms that the client is experiencing. If the survivor seems able to understand my explanation, I will explain very simply the flight/fight sequence of emergency responding, and where I see their symptoms relating to this. I find that survivors are often greatly relieved when given this information. It does not alleviate their symptoms, but they begin to see them as potentially manageable, as having had survival value, and as making sense in a larger context.

Containment and stabilization require the development of internal and external resources. The establishment of the external support structures necessary to stabilize a client's life is often difficult for psychotherapists to effect directly. Clearly, it is essential that survivors of trauma have a place to live, a source of income, and human contact in their lives.

Work with survivors of political torture is particularly challenging in this regard. These survivors are refugees. Often they do not have legal status and fear being returned to the country where they were brutally mistreated. Frequently they are in the painful process of seeking asylum, which is usually retraumatizing for them. Often they are exploited by employers. The language barrier increases their sense of isolation. Dealing with everyday stresses is much more difficult in a foreign country. In treating these survivors, unlike survivors of other types of trauma, I find myself involved with asylum lawyers, teachers, and social service agencies that work with refugees.

As a psychotherapist I am able to directly influence clients' development of internal resources. During this phase of stabilization and containment, I address the symptoms that are disrupting the survivor's sense of equilibrium, such as flashbacks, insomnia, nightmares, hyperarousal, panic attacks, and psycho-somatic problems. All survivors with whom I have worked man-ifest a certain basic physical and energetic organization, referred to as a *shock organization*. There is a freezing and immobilization of the diaphragm, making it difficult to inhale fully, but even more important, impossible to exhale fully. Gen-erally, there is a constriction of the tissue, especially at the base of the skull and in the sacrum. The energy in the body is drawn up out of the legs and feet and inward, away from the extremi-ties to the center of the body. Cold hands and feet are the result. Survivors of political torture I have treated especially seem to experience cold in their lower legs and feet (and feel cold to the touch). Depending on the type and extent of the trauma, there may also be a lack of tissue tone and a general collapse in the body. I observed this in two survivors of torture I worked with in El Salvador (Eckberg, 1997a, 1997b).

Basically, the purpose of somatic work is to restore equilibri-um in the body by addressing the physical and energetic under-pinnings of the shock organization, and thus intervening directly with the distressing symptoms. In this way survivors of trauma can begin to feel in charge of their bodies once again.

Somatic work is essential before beginning to renegotiate and reorganize the traumatic material. During this initial phase of building resources, somatic interventions may be used to facili-tate movement in the diaphragm, leading to a fuller breathing pattern—the ability to inhale fully and to "let down" when exhaling. Moving the energy down into the legs and feet, from the interior of the body to the extremities and to the surface, the skin (points of contact); releasing the constriction in the tissue by working with the tensions; and facilitating the movement of energy in general, results in the client feeling more grounded in present reality and sensing his or her strength and capacity for self-support.

The somatic interventions I find helpful in this regard involve basic breath work and grounding. They come from the tradition of bioenergetics. For instance, sitting in your chair, simply put a little pressure on your feet as you inhale. When exhaling, surrender to the outbreath, making sure you exhale all the air. Trauma survivors have difficulty letting down when exhaling; extending the exhale can make a significant difference in their internal state. You can also work on extending the exhale while standing with knees bent, shoulder width apart. You can bend backwards from this position, making an arc, or what bioenergetics calls the stress position. The same work with the breath can be done lying down with the knees up and the soles of the feet on the floor. Then, while lying down make a gentle rocking motion from head to feet. Kicking by bringing the soles down of the feet hard on the floor is also very grounding and helps to expand the breathing.

This is a sample of the somatic interventions I use most frequently; there are numerous others. Hands-on work may also be helpful in assisting a client to stabilize and to experience his or her resources. I might place my hands gently on either side of the client's head, or I hold the client's head in my hands. Hands-on work on the viscera (where most of the shock energy is held), with one hand supporting the lower back, is very effective in opening up space in the abdomen to permit deeper breathing and the movement of energy down into the legs and feet (i.e., grounding).

Another somatic intervention useful at this stage of treatment, which contributes much to the development of an observing ego, is to ask the client to go even deeper into a particular somatic organization—that is, to exaggerate it slowly—and then to come out of the exaggeration. It is done very slowly with the client staying as aware as possible of what is happening. This intervention also builds co-awareness—the capacity to be here (in the present) and to be there (in the past trauma) at the same time. It is particularly useful to help the survivor become aware of how he or she organizes physically when very anxious, at the beginning of a panic attack, when dissociating, or when feeling immobilized and helpless. The client also begins to develop awareness of sensation, so important for the later work of renegotiating the traumatic material.

I also work with survivors at this beginning stage of stabilization by supporting any positive images or memories that come to mind and encouraging the client's awareness of associated bodily feelings. This helps survivors sense their bodies as resources, not just as sources of pain and suffering. During one of her sessions a survivor of childhood torture produced a healing image of herself dancing in the moonlight. Her bodily experience associated with this image served over and over again to help her learn to sense herself as more expansive and fluid. Another client with a history of severe abuse recalled sitting under an elm tree in her yard, one of the few places she felt safe, stroking her cat and watching the ants do their busy work. Embodying this memory provided important moments of relief when renegotiating the traumatic events of her life.

Two clients come to mind who underline for me the value of knowing how to work on a somatic level. One is a survivor of political torture who had previously seen a number of mental health professionals. She felt that no one had understood her. She was reluctant to try therapy again. In her previous therapy she had been flooding with emotion and reliving the trauma, feeling increasingly out of control. She came to me only because she had been told that I knew a different way of approaching her problems than just talking about what had happened to her. The other client, also a survivor of political torture, was barely holding himself together. He had been in psychotherapy before in his native country, when his brother was "disappeared."[1] He also came only because he had been told by his lawyer that I would be able to approach his problems differently, not just talk about them.

I truly do not know what I would have done with these two clients had I not had the expertise to work on a physical level. I told them that they did not have to talk about what had happened to them. I told them that since I had their testimony from their attorneys (both were in the process of seeking asylum), I knew basic facts of what they had lived through. I assured them that at some point it would be important for us to talk about this, but it would happen in their time and at their pace. Initially, what I was going to do was to help them to feel better.

I began working with their symptoms using somatic interventions. These interventions always varied according to what was happening with the client at that time or even in that particular session. But overall the emphasis was on helping the client to let down while exhaling, to sense the movement of energy down the body when doing this, to ease the movement of energy downward, to encourage elongation and expansiveness in the tissue, and facilitate parasympathetic activity.

Each survivor told me how much he or she did not want to come to the sessions the first few times. After only a few sessions, both clients said that they were beginning to believe that I could help them. Their symptoms began to improve, especially when they practiced the somatic work at home to help them control their symptoms. Both began to talk on their own about the traumatic events, while staying grounded in their bodily experience.

## PHASE TWO:
### RENEGOTIATION, REORGANIZATION, AND INTEGRATION

Survivors of torture have experienced the ultimate in loss of control over their own lives, their own bodies. All survivors of shock trauma have experienced the terror associated with loss of control; it is inherent in the shock experience. Thus, it is important to realize that control is everything to a survivor.

When survivors talk about their traumatic experiences, it is important that they do not relive them and feel out of control and helpless once again, thereby being retraumatized. A survivor needs to understand that acknowledging the feelings and the physiology related to the trauma does not bring back the original trauma itself, and the violence and helplessness associated with it. By intervening directly on the physical and energetic levels of experience (as well as the cognitive and emotional levels), survivors can experience being in charge of their bodily responses while renegotiating and integrating the traumatic events. Keeping the retelling of the trauma story anchored in bodily experience slows the process down, so that more and more detail is included, and gives the client some distance from the experience. Grounding the telling of the trauma story in sensation keeps the survivor connected to present reality and to the therapist. It results in a natural pacing in which the client leads, sets the pace, and is in control of the process. Thus, the survivor is able to reorganize traumatic experience neurophysiologically, as well as emotionally and cognitively, and eventually to establish a coherent, personal narrative, a work that extends throughout the whole course of therapy.

Research and clinical data indicate that traumatic events are remembered primarily in the unconscious mind as somatosensory experience or as implicit memory, and that it is the associated abnormal psychophysiology that drives the symptoms of PTSD.[2] A somatic psychotherapeutic approach offers a way of intervening directly on the biological level in order to restructure the traumatic material to make implicit memory explicit memory. Focus on sensation provides a doorway to the unconscious mind where the potential for deep restructuring and healing lies. Grounding all experience in sensation also allows the client to enter the altered states associated with shock trauma in a controlled manner. Reentering these altered states of mind (state-dependent memory) is necessary in reassociating dissociated memory fragments and in repatterning destructive traumatic responses. The somatic interventions of breath work, grounding, and sensate focusing, used to address symptoms and help stabilize clients, are also useful in this process of renegotiating traumatic events.

Levine (1991,1997) offers a refined and direct method of intervening on the biological level to restructure the traumatic material and make implicit memory explicit memory. In this process cognitive restructuring occurs concurrently with the restructuring of primitive brainstem bodily responses. This way of working gradually destructures traumatic reactions, which are maladaptive neuromuscular patterns underlying PTSD symptomatology. It then restructures these patterns by restoring what was lost in the traumatic event—the basic defensive and orienting responses. Responses to the trauma that lie uncompleted in the nervous system are "unfrozen" and allowed to complete. Innate biological resources overwhelmed at the time of the trauma are re-stored, as is a sense of mastery—the feeling that one is once again able to exert some control over one's body, one's life.

Levine introduces a number of principles that are important in renegotiating traumatic material. The first is the idea of titration. During a shock trauma event a tremendous amount of energy is compressed in the nervous system. Sudden release of this energy results in an explosion of intense emotion and physiological arousal. This is not healing for the victim, but is retraumatizing. Titration (a term borrowed from chemistry) means that only a very small amount of energy is released at a time, allowing body sensations and emotions to be assimilated so that the nervous system can adjust to each level of excitation. This is possible when the retelling remains grounded in bodily experience. If a survivor begins to activate physiologically to the point of becoming anxious and afraid, then the therapist can slow down the process by bringing the client's awareness to her breath, or by asking the client to focus attention on one particular sensation.

This gradual, titrated tracking of sensate, perceptual experience and the associated images, emotions, and thoughts allows for the reassociation of memory fragments. In my experience with this approach, I invariably find a wider and wider expansion of the event, with more and more details gradually being reassociated as we keep each piece of the experience anchored in bodily experience. For instance, if a survivor says, "I am feeling afraid," I would ask, "Where in your body do you feel the fear?" The client might respond, "Right here in my chest." I might ask, "Just what does that fear in your chest feel like?" Client: "Oh, a fluttering, a tightness, a pounding in my heart." Describing in detail or "fleshing out" an experience slows the process down, gives the client some distance, and helps the client to enter the same state of mind occurring at the time of the trauma, allowing fragments of the traumatic memory to reassociate.

This "slow motion" process also opens space for overcoupled trauma responses to uncouple or disassociate, for thwarted defensive and orienting responses to complete, and for moving through tonic immobility or freezing. *Overcoupling* (Levine, 1997) is a term used to refer to the overassociation of sensations, emotions, thoughts, and behaviors related to the traumatic experience: the idea that "all roads lead to the trauma." A classic example of this is a panic attack. In a panic attack one sensation couples with another, then with a thought, then with an emotion, and so on in rapid succession. Uncoupling this chain of experiential events requires slowing the process down, what Levine calls "the taffy-pull"—focusing for a long time on just one sensation, making space for new information to come in. Or the client may be asked to slowly go back and forth between one sensation and another, or one sensation and an emotion, or a sensation and an image.

A client began treatment with me because her panic attacks were feeling increasingly out of control and incapacitating. Initially I worked to help her gain some sense of control over what was happening in her body by teaching her how to let down on the outbreath and how to ground by directing the movement of energy down into her feet. Careful tracking of the sequence of her experience during the panic attacks brought it into her conscious awareness, helping her to feel more in charge of what was happening. It also opened the door to the unconscious substructure driving the panic attacks. Through her exploration, a complex network of associations was made, involving separation anxiety and fear of death, fueled by the fact that both of her parents were Holocaust survivors, while most family members perished.

The survivor of political torture referred to above, who had been tortured by soldiers and then retraumatized by immigration officials, ran at the sight of a man in uniform, manifesting an overcoupling between the impulse to flee and the sight of uniforms. In his treatment process we worked to uncouple his terror from the sight of uniforms and to reassociate his impulses to run (to flee) with his original traumatic experience.

Innate biological responses to threat involve orienting responses and defensive responses. Orienting responses consist of looking around to locate the source of danger. Defensive responses may be very specific to a particular event, but, in general, include physiological arousal, running, pushing away, hitting, kicking, and blocking. When these responses are thwarted, they remain uncompleted in the nervous system. The last-ditch stand of the organism (human or animal), when these life-saving defenses fail, is freezing or tonic immobility. This response may be adaptive when escape is impossible. But when it becomes a habitual/patterned way of responding to threat, it is incapacitating.

Underlying the freezing response are the flight/fight and other orienting and defensive responses, which were in preparation prior to the freezing. Knowing what is happening when a client goes into immobility is essential. If the therapist understands this state and is able to stay in contact with the client, helping him to move through the freezing, the defensive and orienting responses will emerge. Mirroring back to the client what you see happening on a body level is important in maintaining contact: "I see that your eyes are fluttering; now your breath becomes more shallow; I notice some trembling in your arms and hands."

Fundamental to this process is uncoupling the fear or terror from the freezing response. It is essential to keep the client grounded in sensate experience, to slow the process down when necessary, and to encourage blocked defensive and orienting responses, felt as micromovements, to come through. It is important to note that all uncompleted defensive and orienting responses emerge organically from the client's own process. To impose movements on the client is not what I am referring to here. An example of imposing a response would be to tell a client to hit or to push when he or she was feeling immobilized. In contrast, by supporting the client in noting sensory experience and following bodily micromovements, the thwarted flight/fight defensive and orienting responses emerge and are gradually completed and restored.

A survivor of childhood torture, at critical moments in our work together, would become quite immobile except for microscopic rocking movements. I would ask her to notice these micromovements. At first she would freeze completely and say that she could not pay attention to this. Slowly, over time, she was able to focus on these small movements. Then, it was possible for her to allow them to grow into a full rocking motion. As she did this, her fists would clench and she would want to scream and to hit. I surmised that in her tortured childhood, when she had to learn to inhibit her natural rageful responses to her maltreatment, she frequently engaged in rocking behavior.

At first these tiny impulses were constricted each time she felt them in therapy. But eventually she could allow them to move through to the point where she could make hitting and pushing movements and even release her inhibited scream. The restoration of her capacity to protest gradually changed her life. She has become much more able to assert herself in interpersonal interactions.

A client was experiencing body memories associated with a childhood memory of a sadistic punishment. She experienced the sensations as physically painful. After working through the memory and uncoupling the terror and immobility from the sensations (which took many sessions), she said with amazement, when she experienced the same sensations, "Why, they are just sensations; they are not really painful."

Too much intensity is fundamental to the shock trauma experience. The life energy itself easily becomes associated (overcoupled) with anxiety and fear. Sensing one's own aliveness, one's vitality, is then experienced as threatening. Uncoupling (separating) the feeling of terror from the feeling of being intensely alive is an essential part of the treatment. One survivor of severe abuse, who is probably highly energetic and intense by nature, feels frightened of her own aliveness, her own excitement. She finds ways to dampen her excitement and her enthusiasm to avoid the feelings of terror that accompany these states.

In renegotiating traumatic material, a survivor must be able to draw on positive experiences (resources). It is essential that the survivor move between trauma-related physiology, affects, and images, and healing and resourceful bodily states, affects, and images. Two additional concepts from Levine's work speak to this phenomenon: the trauma vortex and the healing vortex. The *trauma vortex* includes all the traumatic reactions involved during the original trauma. Initially there is much more energy in the trauma vortex than in the healing vortex. There is a tremendous pull to enter this pool of undigested and uninte- grated trauma-related experience, resulting in the familiar symptomatology of posttraumatic reactions such as hyper- arousal, terror, flashbacks, and reenactments.

Levine's work recognizes that the nervous system operates according to what Akhter Ahsen (1973) refers to as the "law of bipolarity." He proposes that the seeds of what he calls the *heal- ing vortex* exist and will emerge in the work when the traumat- ic material is carefully tracked and grounded in sensory experience. The client's unconscious mind tends to weave back and forth between the horror of the trauma and the healing resources, which the deep recesses of the unconscious mind itself provides. This pendulum effect of moving from the traumatic material to healing images and parasympathetic responses and then back to the traumatic material is more easily achieved when the traumatic event is a single incident, such as an acci- dent. When the trauma is more complicated, as in repeated events or in a whole childhood of abuse, establishing a healing vortex requires more interventions by the therapist. For instance, I may suggest that a survivor pause and take a breath, surrendering fully to the outbreath, or I may introduce a heal- ing image and the associated bodily state that emerged from the client's own work earlier in the treatment process: "Bring to mind your memory of how strong and powerful your legs felt when you were skiing." Or I say, "Can you remember the image of you and Gloria dancing together as a child and how free you felt? What are you aware of in your body as you see this?"

The movie "Fearless," about the traumatic effects of an air- plane crash, provides an excellent example of the experience of being in each of these vortexes. After the plane crash, the hero is portrayed as stuck in the core of the healing vortex—he feels "fearless," and on a spiritual high. Later, he is struggling in the core of the trauma vortex, feeling overwhelmed by traumatic responses that relate to the shocking event. In his work as an architect he is consumed by the urge to draw vortexes.

According to Levine there is a tendency to swing from the periphery of one vortex to the periphery of the other, or from the core of one to the core of the other. In the renegotiation process, when experience remains grounded in sensation, a survivor generally begins at the periphery of the traumatic content, bringing in peripheral healing components. The tendency is to move closer and closer to the core of the traumatic event while bringing in more and more dramatic healing images and bodily experiences. As survivors move to the core of the traumatic memory, the corresponding healing responses become more spiritual and archetypal. Many times I have felt a sense of awe at what a client's unconscious mind has provided as a balance to the horrific event being renegotiated.

My work with a survivor of political torture provides a rather uncomplicated example of this vacillation between the two vortexes. He was captured and horribly tortured for months by the military in his country of origin. He was referred to me by his asylum attorney. When preparing his testimony with her, he would repeatedly turn pale, perspire profusely, and "begin to faint." Because of this she would have to stop the process and have him return at a later date. Seven visits to his attorney were necessary for him to relate to her the information required for her to plead his asylum case.

When I began working with him I assured him that he did not have to tell me his story, although at some point he might want to, and that it would be important. I told him that his lawyer had sent me his testimony. I added that we would begin by working to help him to feel better. He manifested classic

PTSD symptoms: insomnia, nightmares, hypervigilance, flash-backs, and panic attacks in which he would begin to shake all over.

I began working with his breathing, with grounding, and with sensory awareness. He stabilized and began to feel more in charge of his bodily responses after only four or five sessions. As we worked somatically, he began to tell me his story sponta-neously, while also relating his sensory experience.

He began at the periphery, telling me about his life in his country long before his torture experience. He would then talk about his life now in the U.S. Gradually he talked more about his life in his own country closer to the time of his captivity. He related tales of friends disappearing, of finding the mutilated bodies of friends and relatives. He would then talk about his arrival in the U.S. and his interrogation by immigration agents. Eventually, he arrived at the core of the trauma vortex—the grizzly details of his torture experience.

Throughout this process his mind would bring in positive memories of his childhood, of supportive relationships in his past and current life. He would refer on his own to parasympa-thetic responses, such as warmth, tingling, or a sense of spa-ciousness at critical moments, or I would encourage this if necessary. After he renegotiated all aspects of his trauma, in-cluding his extensive recovery process after his torture experi-ence, a later attempt to assassinate him, and his escape to the U.S., his symptoms virtually disappeared. He would say to me in Spanish, as he again recounted parts of his experience, "Look at me, look at me, I am telling you what happened and I am not trembling and shaking, I am not afraid."

This survivor was particularly easy to treat, and positive results were achieved in a relatively short time. I believe there are several reasons for this. One is that this survivor is a very strong man, both physically and emotionally. He is also intelligent and well educated. He understood in detail the political situation in his country of origin. He was himself involved in political activity. Clinical data show that survivors of political torture fare much better if they have been political, which provides a context that makes some sense of their mistreatment. Survivors of political torture who manifest the worst symptoms and have the most difficulty recovering are those who are just caught in the cross fire—who are simply in the wrong place at the wrong time. In addition, my impression was that this man had dissociated only somewhat during his torture experience. Research suggests that a moderate amount of dissociation during a traumatic event results in less severe symptomatology than a great deal of dissociation or none at all (van der Kolk, 1996).

The process of renegotiation described above becomes more complex and difficult when the shock trauma events are repetitive and occur at a earlier age. However, the same phenomena are operating and the same principles are applicable whether the trauma is an accident, an experience of torture, or a whole history of child abuse.

## PHASE THREE:
### EXPANSION AND THE CAPACITY TO EXPERIENCE PLEASURE

A survival mode of functioning results in constriction in the body and in experience and activity, resulting in a diminished capacity for pleasure. Overstimulation of the nervous system makes it difficult to relax. Fixation on the trauma because of overcoupling and state-dependent memory also contributes to a pleasureless existence.

I am working with a survivor of political torture whose symptoms of insomnia, flashbacks, and hyperarousal have improved markedly. However, her life is restricted to going to work, to the laundromat, and to the market. When she is home she refuses to join her husband in watching TV or listening to music. She won't accompany him to mass, to weddings, parties, or any social gatherings. She explains to me that to listen to music makes her feel sad, to watch TV she risks feeling upset, and when she is in a group of people she fears something terrible will happen. It reminds her of the funerals in her country of origin or of the groups that gathered when dead bodies were found.

As we speak of this, she sits on the couch with her body tightly constricted, her shoulders almost up to her ears. She notes her position, having achieved some body awareness and insight, and realizes that she is organized in a position of fear. On a cognitive level she knows that she would not be in any danger if she accompanied her husband to these social activities. Yet she is adamant that she will not expand her behavior to include these potentially positive experiences.

She has, however, begun to be open to sensing herself more positively. She goes for a weekly massage from one of the treatment providers at the Healing Center for Survivors of Political Torture. Using what she has learned in her sessions with me, she is able to induce a relaxed, parasympathetic state by working with herself at home. Now, when she is home alone, she takes warm baths and calls friends on the phone instead of sitting immobile doing nothing or constantly cleaning and organizing her house.

Another client, who is in the process of working through the core of her shock trauma experience, was hardly able to hold a positive thought in her mind about her past, present, or future. It was a dramatic example of state-dependent memory: Experiencing the extraordinary painful and terrifying feelings of her traumatic past blocked any access to positive memories or experiences. Then she attended a ten-day vipassana meditation retreat, a practice that encourages one to be open to whatever arises in awareness, without judgment. For the first four days she observed the negativity of her experience—judgments, criticisms, bad memories, painful sensations. On the fifth day, during a walking meditation, she was moved to tears by the long-forgotten pleasurable experience of walking barefoot in wet grass. A flood of positive childhood memories followed, beginning with the shoeless, carefree summers at her family's lake home. This experience also seemed to open a gateway to current pleasure. She was able to enjoy the blueness of the sky, the green trees, the smells of the flowers, and to have positive, hopeful thoughts about the future.

I recently treated a client who barely survived a serious accident involving a high-impact head injury. Embedded in the shock core of her experience was the sense of being unable to stop what was happening—losing control of her bike, being thrown through the air, finding herself totally helpless on the ground, and realizing that she could not stop the pain. During her treatment she returned from a ski trip and began to talk about how positive her experience of skiing had been. I asked her to tell me more and inquired what she was aware of now in her body. Soon she was standing, making the movements of skiing, clearly feeling expansive and filled with pleasure. She was saying, "I can stop, and I can stop. Yes, I can stop." This served as one of many resources helping her to regain a sense of control and allowing her to feel less helpless and more expansive in her life.

In my work with clients, I have learned that helping them to develop their sensory awareness is not only essential in renegotiating and integrating their traumatic experiences, but also is the avenue to a more pleasurable mode of existence. Using the somatic interventions of breathing, grounding, and sensory awareness, I help survivors to enter more relaxed, parasympathetic states, so that they can begin to get enjoy the experiences of pleasure, satisfaction, and humor. I draw on any positive memories of past or current experiences, fleshing them out and expanding them at the sensory level, to help them develop and trust a more expanded sense of self. I find that this leads to an opening of one's self-experience to more than just the trauma— to a gradual expansion of life experience and activity.

## INTEGRATION OF TRAUMATIC MATERIAL AND FORMATION OF A COHESIVE STORY

As the work progresses, the content and affect related to the traumatic event are integrated into a sense of self. Orienting and defensive responses are restored, as well as an increased capacity to modulate arousal in the nervous system. The gap between the pretraumatic and posttraumatic identity closes, and there is more integration between the two.

I once treated a client who had completely lost touch with who she was before the traumatic events of her life occurred. During the course of her therapy, an image emerged of who she had been prior to the trauma. Her positive qualities had been totally forgotten and were unavailable to her.

When the client is finally able to form a cohesive story of a particular traumatic event or a cohesive life story, and to derive meaning from the events, the spiritual level is often activated. The meaning of events begins to be understood at a metaphysical level.

### GRIEVING

Most of the clients with whom I have worked pass through a period of profound grieving as they approach the end of their therapy or of their work on a particular traumatic episode. They seem to grieve for what they lost in the traumatic experience and for what they never had the opportunity to experience. If we are dealing with a whole childhood of abuse, they grieve for the impact that the trauma has had on their entire lives.

When traumatic material is still dissociated, the grieving

cannot occur. Only after the client feels the reality of how the trauma has shaped his or her basic existence does the door to these deep wells of grief seem to open.

A client who survived a near fatal accident experienced profound grief for several months, during her sessions and between sessions. The grief deepened as she slowly integrated the seriousness of the accident and how extensively it had affected her life. The accident had caused no disability; she was in very good health. Thus, there was nothing tangible that she was grieving for.

Another client, who had survived extreme abuse as a teenager and young adult, grieved deeply for at least six months, after about three years of work to integrate these experiences. She had always remembered the facts of the experiences, but had never been able to take in the impact they had had on her life.

## HANDS-ON WORK

The majority of hands-on work that I do is related to support, especially of the head, back, and shoulders. I preface hands-on supportive work with, "I would like to give you a little support . . ." and then say where I will provide the support. I may support the person's head while he is sitting up or lying down. Or I may place my hand on a client's back while she is standing, or under the small of the back while he is lying down. I may touch the client's foot with mine while she is in an altered state with her eyes closed to let her know that I am there and available to her. I also use touch to assist in grounding the client's energy by holding the head, with the client lying down, the feet, or the hands.

Release of tension or energy blocks in the body is another reason to do hands-on work. Placing my hands on an area that is constricting energy flow often relieves the constriction and enhances the expansion of the tissue in the area. For instance, I may place my hands on the client's neck, abdomen and lower back, or diaphragm. Levine (personal communication) emphasizes opening what he calls the four diaphragms by placing one's hands on the periphery of these areas. To begin, I place my hands on the client's temples and wait until I sense some expansion in the tissue. Usually I feel that the skin is coming out to meet my hands. Next, I place my hands on the outside of the shoulders and upper arms and wait for the expansion. Then, I place my hands on the person's sides at the level of the regular diaphragm. Finally, I put my hands on the periphery of the person's pelvis. This is very grounding and facilitates the restoration of the wave of energy that moves down the body. This wave of energy is greatly disturbed by shock states related to trauma.

I find it extremely important to use touch to provide nonverbal contact when working through preverbal, early infancy, or fetal trauma. The client often needs to experience the therapist's presence through sensation and the lower brainstem, rather than verbally or through the cerebral cortex.

I am quite aware of the debate over whether or not touch is appropriate in psychotherapy.[3] Touch clearly has different meanings for different patients. There are some clients I would never touch; for instance, clients for whom it would complicate the transference and who have little observing ego. One must be sure that the touch will contribute to the treatment process, rather than elicit strong regressive feelings or sexual impulses, or overwhelm the client with too much activation. The touch must be therapeutic and must not be based in the therapist's own needs. It is also important for the therapist to realize that touching may complicate and intensify the countertransference (Hilton, 1997). Thus, staying finely attuned to my own response when touching a client is central to using touch in a therapeutic manner.

# Chapter Three

———— ✦ ————

# TRANSFERENCE AND SOCIETAL TRAUMA

Much has been written about the clinical relationship—the personal interactions that transpire during the therapeutic process. My intention in this chapter is to point out how much more intense and complex these relationships become when shock trauma is part of the clinical picture. I have included a cautionary note about the risks of secondary traumatization for the therapist when working with traumatized persons. Related to this is the secondary traumatization and the interpersonal acting out of traumatic violence that can occur when a whole society suffers shocking events. We then see the society degenerating into individuals living out the roles of victims or perpetrators, with horrifying consequences.

## TRANSFERENCE AND COUNTERTRANSFERENCE

The therapist-client relationship creates an intersubjective field (Stolorow, Atwood, and Brandchaft, 1994) and a somatic responsiveness between the two persons. Their interaction re-creates the past in present-day relationship. The therapist must be able to engage these transference/countertransference feelings and observe, contain, and process them without becoming enmeshed in reenacting them.[1] Healing comes where the therapist disconfirms the client's schemas of meaning and helps the client to integrate the past horror of trauma with present experience. Although I subscribe to the intersubjective perspective, I have found it useful in teaching to talk about transference and countertransference separately.

## Transference

Transference specific to the trauma almost always occurs. When painful traumatic material is brought into the present in the treatment setting, there is a re-creation of dissociated aspects of self and object representations. Unconscious or dissociated trauma reenactments often involve interpersonal experiences and invite others (therapists) to respond in complementary ways.

A client with whom I have very good rapport and a high level of trust is a survivor of early infantile and childhood abuse by her mother. After years of no contact, she met with her mother and with another therapist. Then she was hesitant to come to her next session with me. She showed up with terror in her eyes and kept me at a physical distance for most of the session, before recognizing that she was afraid of being overwhelmed and engulfed by me, as she had felt years ago by her mother. After four-and-a-half years of therapy, another highly traumatized client still sits on one side of the room in my fairly spacious office and insists that I sit on the other side, keeping as much physical distance between us as possible.

Survivors may see the therapist as a threat and tend to expect the worst from their therapist. In the therapist and even the therapist's office they see a threatening force that can harm them. This may not be a cognitive process. I have two doors to my office, and several clients have commented how relieved they are that I cannot sit between them and a way out of the room. Unlike my clients who do not suffer from shock trauma, survivors are very sensitive to any noise outside the office. Two clients expressed concern about what was behind a folding door in my office. Both wanted to know if it was a door to the outside (i.e., could someone come in?).

The therapist may be seen as a violator of boundaries. This might manifest as difficulty establishing boundaries or as the need for very rigid boundaries. Because of the intensity of the shock energy, boundary violations are more likely to occur with survivors of shock trauma, who try to pull the therapist into a traumatic reenactment. One of the most common boundary violations is an attempt to "love the patient into health" by extending the length of sessions, being overly available by phone between sessions, scheduling frequent emergency sessions, or engaging in dual relationships. Many survivors have never had a close connection with anyone. It is not unusual for such clients to want the relationship with the therapist to broaden into a friendship.

The therapist may be seen as a betrayer. As trust develops, survivors become most afraid and may retreat or even leave therapy. Many therapists have had a client do something to create distance just when we sense the client is beginning to trust us. This pattern is exhibited even more intensely by trauma survivors.

The therapist may also be perceived as an interrogator or judge, resulting in feelings of rejection, humiliation, and degradation. A woman with dissociated identity disorder whom I treated for years developed a characteristic pattern of behavior at the beginning of her treatment, which exemplifies both of the above transferences. After a session in which we were quite engaged and I felt that she had let me in, one of her "alters" would call and unload her anger on me for "treating her like a puppet," by trying to control her and manipulate her. I soon realized that the sessions in which I asked more questions and in which she responded more to me apparently left her feeling invaded and would result in her angry phone calls.

Another transferential perspective is for the client to see the therapist as a victim of his lethal self. The survivor believes himself to be evil, malignant, and lethal to all who become close to him. He fears that the therapist will die, be destroyed, or meet a tragic fate. It is a form of the magical thinking of the child, but it feels absolutely real to the survivor. I am treating a client who felt this very strongly at one point in our relationship. She feared that I would be killed in some bizarre way or that I would become ill and even die because of my closeness to her. Much work with her child alters was necessary to change her outlook.

A very common transference manifested by trauma survivors is the determination not to become dependent on the therapist. Independence and the belief that one can only rely on oneself is an important part of their belief system. Allowing oneself to trust that the therapist can be there for you results in feeling too vulnerable. Thus, the only option is to deny the importance of the therapist and one's own vulnerability.

Control is everything to the survivor, and some need to feel that they are in control of their sessions. I find ways to allow this, while at the same time feeling that I am still in charge of what is happening in the room. I do this by maintaining a strong frame around the therapy and a strong presence in the room.

One client has a childhood history abuse; she was also traumatized in a spiritual community as an adult. She had spent three years feeling totally out of control and hanging on the edge of psychosis. When she came to me, she insisted on bringing her agenda for each session written on a piece of paper. The agenda was repetitive and could have been boring for me had I not realized the deeper meaning of this behavior. It was a long time before she was able to relinquish some of her control to allow more intervention on my part. Fortunately she is smart, has some observing ego, and has a sense of humor, and we could joke with each other about her control issues. But I also let her know that I understood her need to feel in control after so long feeling out of control and overwhelmed in her life.

Survivors have often experienced traumatic loss of loved ones through death or betrayal. This may manifest as an extreme fear of loss of the therapist. One of my clients feared I would be killed every time I left town. Her fear was so strong that for a time it would consume her whenever I took time off. Gradually, she worked this through.

It is important to help such a client come to terms with the unpredictability of life. It is also necessary to help the patient understand that now, in present-day reality, loss of the therapist will not shatter her.

Survivors and therapists alike can become addicted to the exploration of traumatic experiences. The client feels overwhelmed under such circumstances and may begin to feel unsafe in the therapist's office. Then the client may view the therapist as the perpetrator who is making her relive painful memories. Of course, the therapist may be cast in the role of perpetrator without such a dynamic occurring. However, it is much more likely to happen when the trauma is being cathartically relived.

In dealing with the transference, it is crucial that the therapist remain grounded in his or her own body and in the present. I am always attentive to my own breathing and my own somatic responsiveness. Awareness of the felt sense in my own body also alerts me to cues about the transference occurring. I am able to use the somatic interventions that facilitate grounding during the session and between sessions. While just sitting in my chair, I am able to move energy down to my legs and feet while just lengthening my exhale. This is very subtle and not visible to the client. When I am working somatically with clients, I do the grounding work with them, both to be supportive of them and to keep myself well grounded.

There are two somatic interventions I find useful in helping survivors to develop a more observing ego of their own transference. One of these is simply to ask the client what he is aware of in his body when he is organized in a transferential position. Because sensory awareness is a direct doorway to the unconscious mind, this frequently leads to a chain of associations that connects the client's feelings toward the therapist to the client's past. Thus, the client is able to arrive at this insight on his own, without interpretation by me.

Another helpful intervention is to ask the client to intensify how she is organized physically and then to release the intensification. I ask the client to do this very slowly with awareness of all levels of experience (sensation, image, behavior, emotions, and thoughts). This often facilitates a flood of associations, which ultimately bring insight to the client's transference. Again, this happens without actual interpretation by me. Usually it results in the client being more conscious of unconscious patterns of relating to the therapist. The somatic interventions of sensory awareness and grounding also help enormously in working with transference by keeping the client anchored to present-day reality, mitigating some of the intensity of the feeling and the tendency to attribute it to the current situation.

## COUNTERTRANSFERENCE

Therapists working with trauma survivors experience a wide range of feelings, which may be very intense.[2] They may feel guilt, rage, dread, grief, or shame. They may feel overwhelmed; they may use the defenses of numbing, denial, and avoidance. There is also a tendency for these professionals to isolate themselves from those around them and to gravitate toward others doing the same kind of work. Therapists working with survivors are vulnerable to empathic strain or compassion fatigue, i.e., difficulty remaining in empathic connection with the survivor.

It is very important for therapists to acknowledge the feelings elicited in them in their work with survivors. We must normalize our reactions the same way that we normalize our clients' responses to traumatic events, i.e., that these are normal responses to abnormal events. To experience physiological and emotional reactions is normal and necessary in achieving empathy with a client. If we do not have some reaction, we are unable to become attuned to the client's experience, which is essential in work with trauma.

Remaining attuned to my own somatic experience is a crucial aid in helping me to recognize my own feelings and reactions in my work with survivors. Staying aware of my breath and my feet on the floor ground me in the present, so that I am less likely to be swept away by a countertransferential response. I often use the technique of exaggerating how I am organized while visualizing a client. By focusing on the associations that arise as I do so, I gain insight into my own experience of the person. This is an intervention I have used a great deal in supervising interns and other therapists in their work with trauma survivors. I am often amazed at how quickly this attention to one's bodily experience produces important insights into previously inexplicable reactions. This somatic awareness brings into the conscious mind feelings and thoughts hitherto unrecognized and unacknowledged.

For example, a client was recently retraumatized by a real-life event (a natural disaster). I was out of town at the time and could not respond to her call immediately, although I had a therapist on call for me. After my return I began to receive angry phone calls, suicide threats, and refusals to keep her appointments with me (she also had transportation difficulties at the time). My response was to stay calm and contained. However, visualizing her and exaggerating my somatic organization, I quickly got in touch with feelings of helplessness and anger. I realized that I was feeling exactly as she did when being abused by a relative without her parents recognizing what was happening. I also became aware of how my responses were tying into my own traumatic past and influencing how I was responding to her. By working with myself somatically to disorganize my constricted, collapsed, self-diminishing physical stance and grounding myself in the present, I was able to take a firmer position with her, while at the same time remaining empathic with how devastated she was feeling.

Although it is essential to acknowledge our affective reactions, it is also important to remember that any affective response may evolve into a countertransferential response that can disrupt the therapy. I find it useful to differentiate between countertransference that is normative and universal and that which is personal. The former includes reactions that most persons would have in listening to survivors' stories. The latter exists when our own issues become activated. Sometimes it can be very difficult to perceive the difference between our own issues being activated and suffering from secondary trauma.

Basic countertransference reactions can be organized into three main categories. The first involves withdrawal. The therapist pulls back, "numbs out," avoids certain material, becomes detached, or actually dissociates from the client. The second reaction is overinvolvement. This includes enmeshment, overidentification with the client, and over-emphasis on the traumatic material. The therapist falls into the role of rescuer, failing to keep clear boundaries. Third, the therapist may simply experience disequilibrium. Emotional and physiological reactions to the traumatic material throw the therapist off balance. He or she is unable to stay present and respond appropriately to the client. It is not uncommon for a therapist to focus only on the exploration of traumatic memories. In that case the therapist and client alike end up feeling overwhelmed and helpless.

I emphasize again that in my experience, somatic awareness

and the somatic work I referred to above are important tools in recognizing how the therapist is responding to the client. These tools help in maintaining one's balance in the tumultuous back and forth exchange, on so many levels, between the client and therapist. I find that it takes years for somatic awareness to become automatic for the therapist, without requiring an ongoing conscious effort. But, beginning therapists will also find it extremely useful.

## SECONDARY TRAUMATIZATION

Secondary traumatization is defined as the painful and disruptive psychophysiological effects of knowing trauma victims or hearing about traumatic events. Mental health professionals, police officers, paramedics, rescue workers, social workers, child protection workers—anyone who works with or is in close contact with survivors of traumatic events can experience secondary traumatization. Its effects are distinguished from similar concepts, such as countertransference or burnout. Crucial to the definition of secondary traumatization is that the symptoms manifested by those suffering from it are basically the same as in the survivors themselves.[3]

The symptoms of secondary traumatization seen in those in close contact with survivors are directly related to the symptoms of posttraumatic stress disorder listed in the *DSM-IV*:

1. Intrusive imagery related to the client's traumatic experiences, such as repetitious thoughts, preoccupation with mental pictures of the traumatic events, and nightmares.

2. Avoidant responses to anything related to the survivor's traumatic experiences, such as movies, TV, the newspaper, or avoiding traumatic material in the course of psychotherapy.

3. Blunted affect and numbing, usually experienced as gradual distancing from one's own feelings and sensations, resulting in distancing oneself from the survivor as well.

4. Physiological arousal: hyperarousal, hypervigilance, feeling overwhelmed and stressed out, disorganized and disoriented so that it is difficult to make even minor decisions or to accomplish everyday tasks. One may also experience distressing emotions like fear, terror, rage, helplessness, and confusion.

5. Somatic complaints, which could be anything from actual illness to undiagnosed pain.

6. Addictive or compulsive behavior of any kind, including overwork—a very common symptom.

7. Sleep disturbances, which always compound and aggravate the other problems.

8. Preoccupation with the safety of oneself and loved ones, such as a decrease in so-called "risky" behavior, overconcern for the safety of one's children, preoccupation with strange noises or with locking doors.

9. Counterphobic behavior, manifested as exposing oneself to danger. An example of this is the behavior of my own daughter when suffering from secondary traumatization while living in El Salvador. A man had pulled a gun on her on the street. After she had initially done the correct thing (yell and attract attention) she turned and followed him.

10. A tendency to become isolated, to talk less to family and friends about one's work in an effort to protect

them. We may gravitate more toward colleagues and conferences.

11.  Dissociation "spacing out"; not present for clients or others.

12.  Feelings of helplessness, related to the survivor's feelings of helplessness, and exacerbated by being in the role of helper and by the intensity and intransigence of the survivor's symptoms.

13.  Driven behavior and an inability to relax, manifested primarily as overwork in an attempt to handle the hyperarousal and/or to feel omnipotent, to avoid feelings of helplessness.

14.  Disruption of cognitive schemas. Being exposed to the survivor's traumatic experiences disrupts our cognitive organization of how the world is or ought to be. Realizing the evil in the world, the horror human beings can perpetrate on one another, challenges one's mind-set that the world is basically fair and just and safe.

Thus, secondary traumatization will result in impaired functioning. However, the impairment tends to be acute, rather than chronic, meaning that those affected recover quickly, compared to those suffering from primary PTSD. Because of my own trauma history and the fact that I am always, at some level, dealing with my own symptoms of primary PTSD, I may also suffer at times with the effects of secondary traumatization. I will discuss later how I manage the impact of this on me, as well as the impact of my own trauma. Thus, the examples I will give of secondary traumatization are not my personal experiences, but the experiences I have observed in other helping professionals.

As director of the Healing Center for Survivors of Political Torture, I helped the psychotherapists and body workers deal with the impact this work was having on them. I constantly encouraged these treatment providers to use the somatic interventions they know so well and were using with the survivors. Working with their own breathing and grounding their energy both during and outside of sessions was crucial for them to contain the trauma to which they were exposed and to maintain their own stability. We had a system set up; they were to immediately call me or another treatment provider if they began to feel overwhelmed after sessions with their clients.

Also helpful is that all of these treatment providers were engaged in their own somatic psychotherapy or body work on a regular basis. Perhaps the most challenging aspect, however, was helping the providers deal with the disruption of their cognitive organization of how the world is. We had many discussions about how one can come to grips with the knowledge of so much evil and horror in the world. I found the process related to this to be very individualistic; each provider had to find his or her own way. Support from others seemed to be the most important in helping them to reorganize how they perceived the world.

An example of secondary traumatization, which then triggered a primary full-blown PTSD response, was experienced by a student I was supervising. The student was an intern at the an outpatient clinic and was also seeing survivors of political torture at the Healing Center. She had a tendency to overextend herself and not to know her limits. About a third of her clients were highly traumatized, a large number for an intern. In retrospect, I fault myself for not monitoring her more closely.

I was out of town for about three weeks. When I returned, I learned that she had begun to suffer from some mild PTSD symptoms that seemed related to her work, such as anxiety, insomnia, and feeling overwhelmed. Then her already vulnerable state and some added stress in her personal life resulted in her developing a full-blown PTSD reaction, causing her to take two weeks off.

There is no way to untangle how much of this was secondary trauma and how much was related to her own traumatic past. However, the effects, although dramatic, were fortunately short-lived. Within about three weeks she was functioning reasonable normally, although sobered by her experience. It was also a warning to me to follow therapists that I am supervising more closely.

Two additional examples are even closer to home. My daughter is living and working in El Salvador. During one of my trips to El Salvador to train professionals to work with traumatized individuals and communities, she accompanied me on a trip to a rural community. This was my first visit to El Salvador and, although I speak Spanish, I was not confident that I would understand the rural dialect adequately. My daughter offered to sit in on my first consultation with a woman who had a serious trauma history. As the woman's story began to unfold, I could feel that my daughter, who was sitting next to me, was becoming activated. It was something I was sensing and hearing in her breathing; there were no obvious outward manifestations. I should have suggested that she leave, but she stayed for the entire two-hour interview.

Afterward she engaged in several healing activities. She immediately went outside and wrote a beautiful poem about the woman, discharging some of the energy that had built up in her. For the rest of the day she acted and looked fine. But as soon as we arrived at her house in San Salvador and we were alone she wept and wept. Over and over she exclaimed, "What a terrible life she has had!" Once again she was discharging the excess energy held in her body since the consultation. We talked some about her experience. She soon settled down. She gained a new respect for the possible impact on her of living and working in a country highly traumatized by a cruel and inhuman civil war.

A year or so later I began receiving phone calls from my daughter, often in the middle of the night. She sounded like someone with full-blown PTSD, although she does not have her own shock trauma history. She was experiencing panic and shortness of breath. She was often unable to sleep, and then she would panic about the possible effects on her work. She felt totally overwhelmed; everything seemed as though it was too much. Fortunately, this was shortly before Christmas, and she was coming home for the holidays.

When she returned, I learned that she had been doing an evaluation of a project for the Catholic church. The project consisted of finding children abandoned by their guerrilla parents when they went off to fight and placing them with family or foster parents. Her job was to interview the children and their parents or foster parents. Thus, she was spending seven days a week in the *campo* (countryside) talking to people about their traumatic experiences during the war. She had become completely drawn into and consumed by the process.

We did a good deal of healing work while she was home: hands-on body work, work with her breathing to open it up, processing her feelings by talking about her experiences. She got a lot of sleep and regular exercise. Within two weeks she returned to El Salvador in reasonably good shape. She was relaxed and grounded and sleeping normally. Once again I saw the danger of exposing oneself to the traumatic wounds of others without adequate training in keeping one's boundaries and without adequate support (she had no one in El Salvador with whom she could discuss her experiences). It also brought home to me the acute, rather than chronic nature of secondary traumatization, especially if the person does not have his or her own trauma history.

What is important in preventing and dealing with secondary traumatization? Research indicates that professionals with less experience and training are more vulnerable to its effects (McCann and Pearlman, 1990; Pearlman and Saakvitne, 1994). Support from participation in professional activities, training, and support groups is very important in maintaining one's stability. It is crucial to be able to talk with others about this work. It helps to discharge the intense energy associated with exposure to shock trauma events and ensures that one does not begin to feel isolated with one's experience. It is also important to participate in a variety of activities other than trauma-related work. Those who do this work have a tendency to constrict their lives (as the survivors themselves do). Note the example above of how my daughter became consumed by her work.

I believe it is safe to conclude that a person who has a trauma history is more vulnerable to secondary trauma. But this is not the case when one has worked through one's own personal trauma and faced one's own demons. Also, this effect diminishes with experience in the field. Minimizing other stresses in your life is also important. Knowing your own limits and setting boundaries is a significant determinant of maintaining one's stability when working with survivors. To give up one's naivete and reorganize one's consciousness to incorporate the knowledge of such horror in the world is challenging at best and may feel devastating to some. It interferes with one's assumptions of personal invulnerability and of the world as meaningful and comprehensible. To do this work requires knowing that humans have the capacity for utmost evil.

How does one acquire such a mindset? In my experience, each person must find his or her own way. I dealt with this basic struggle when I was twenty years old, long before I began to work with survivors. My personal trauma brought me face to face with evil. One of the ways that I integrated the knowledge of evil in my world was to read about it. I devoured books about the Holocaust, Native Americans, and slavery in an attempt to find some understanding of it all. When I began working with trauma survivors I had already grappled with this question and was never knocked off balance by the stories of horror. For me, it continues to be important to have a spiritual belief system to help me, too.

In doing this work, constantly examine how the work affects your personal identity, your view of the world, spirituality, relationships, dreams, and emotional responsiveness to others. What happens to your sense of safety in the world? How vulnerable to harm do you feel? How hypervigilant are you? How adrenalized are you?

If you find yourself feeling spacy, constricted, adrenalized, or overwhelmed, it is helpful to intensify and release the way you are organized physically to undo the shock organization in your body. This will get the energy wave moving again and establish more parasympathetic activity. One can only stay connected to one's client by being connected to oneself. In general, I stress how crucial it is to stay grounded when doing this work. "Staying grounded" means that one feels connected to oneself and to the ground—that there is some expansiveness in the body tissue, rather than constriction. One's breathing is open, and there is a fluidity and movement of energy through the body.

To ensure that I stay grounded and stabilized, I do a number of things: I meditate for an hour in the morning; I go to a health club where I exercise and detoxify in the sauna and the hot tub; and develop very good boundaries in my contact with survivors. Instead of feeling tired at the end of a day, I often feel more energized than at the beginning.

Finally, I wish to stress that working with seriously traumatized people can be very rewarding. I continue to feel in awe of the resiliency of the human spirit. The creative ways in which people manage to survive never cease to amaze me. The human capacity for recovery is truly heartening.

## TRAUMATIZATION OF A SOCIETY

The effects of traumatization of a whole society parallel the effects of shock trauma on an individual. As with an individual one can observe in a whole society the following: denial, dissociation, reenactment, impunity, lack of integration of traumatic material, destruction of identity, and the breaking of connections. I base my observations on what I have read, what I have heard from survivors of political oppression with whom I have worked, and on my own experience in El Salvador, a highly traumatized country.

## DENIAL

There is a tendency for members of a society who have lived through a time of atrocity to refuse to believe what has happened. Denial, a much underrated defense, is very useful when it comes to survival. Not to speak of a traumatic event is a way to avoid being retraumatized, both for an individual and for society as a whole. However, if a society, like an individual, is to heal, there is a need to face the truth of what happened, to talk about it. Some children of Holocaust survivors say that their parents never talked about the Holocaust. In El Salvador many refer to the twelve years of the brutal civil war as "the lost decade," meaning that there is a strong tendency to talk as though it never happened. Friends who lived through "the dirty war" in Argentina talk about the shallowness in that society since that period. Just like an individual, a society has to face the reality of what actually happened. Just like an individual, a society cannot focus on hedonistic materialistic pursuits, and superficial interests to prevent the truth from surfacing and being dealt with.

I also observed this in China. There was a powerful superficial, ugly capitalism and a greed mentality that seemed to motivate people. After reading numerous books on the Maoist years, I found it mind-boggling to see the society thriving on this surface level, as though the horror that had transpired not so many years earlier had never occurred.

## DISSOCIATION

Dissociation manifests on a societal level in two basic ways. One is the tendency for the whole society to split into victims and perpetrators, acting out the split in meaningless violence. Reich (1970) was perhaps the first to address how individuals split off the victim part and/or the perpetrator part of themselves and project it onto others. On a societal level, one sees phenomena such as the persecution of the Jews in Nazi Germany, the atrocities committed by American soldiers in Vietnam, and many forms of genocide around the world.

Another form of dissociation in society is for the members to actually dissociate, rather than just to deny parts of what happened. The result is that the society does not remember the horror of what happened. Just as an individual needs to integrate traumatic material, a whole society must do the same if it is to heal on a societal level. It has taken about fifty years for the Germans to integrate the horror of the Holocaust. More than twenty-five years have passed since the American disaster in Vietnam. Only now are we beginning to really digest this experience and own our role as perpetrator. In America we have not even begun to integrate our role as perpetrator in Central and South America. Numerous books have been written and movies made about these traumatic events, helping to guide societies to integrate into their sense of history the unimaginable, the inconceivable.

## REENACTMENT

Because of denial and dissociation, trauma on a societal level continues in the form of violence. Sometimes the violence is organized, as is so often observed when a new government comes into power and soon is repeating the abuses of the past government. Often the violence is just random, as is the case in El Salvador.

One example was reported by a professional who attended one of the workshops I did there. His job took him frequently into the campo (countryside) where he was friends with the people who live there, including ex-guerrillas. One morning when he was waiting on the road for his ride, he was attacked by men he knew to be ex-guerrillas. The members of the community stood by and did not intervene, because of their own fear. He was badly beaten. The attack was without apparent motive.

Having a gun pulled on you on the street is a common event. When this happened to my daughter, she talked about it with people she knew and found that about half of them had had a similar experience.

One is warned in El Salvador not to drive on the highway at night. Armed men block the road and rob or kill those foolish enough to ignore this warning.

One might even hypothesize that in various hot spots around the world, where there is one war after another, one perpetration of genocide after another, an energetic trauma field has been established. Just living in this energy sets the stage for more traumatic events to occur.

## DESTRUCTION OF IDENTITY

Destruction or marked alteration of identity is inevitable when an individual is traumatized. Like an individual, a society is never the same once it has been traumatized. The trauma affects values and norms and the ways individuals in the society think of themselves.

Like individual trauma, societal trauma involves the problem of impunity. In interpersonal trauma, most of the time those who are guilty are never brought to justice. Just as a traumatized individual has much confusion about who is responsible for his or her suffering, a whole society becomes confused. Social and moral values are destroyed, resulting in superficial, materialistic, decadent, and hedonistic behavior.

## BROKEN CONNECTIONS

In individuals who have been traumatized we observe the internal fragmentation between different parts of their experience and the broken attachment bonds with others. Individuals' self-survival takes precedence over species survival; self-survival takes over on a societal level too. When I was in El Salvador I was struck by the alienation among community members. This was especially significant because the country has a long history of strong community orientation. The professionals with whom I interacted worked very much in isolation, whereas before and during the war they had worked closely connected with other professionals. The communities I visited tended to be fragmented and to be looking to outsiders to solve their problems.

For a community to heal and to feel whole again requires community interaction and the rebuilding of social bonds. A few of the professionals with whom I worked were making efforts to rebuild personal connections among community members. They formed support groups and held meetings with community members to educate them about symptoms of posttraumatic stress disorder.

## Healing

In addition to verbal interactions, another powerful form of healing transpires when people interact physically and energetically. As pointed out in earlier chapters, posttraumatic symptomatology is driven primarily by the lower, more primitive parts of the brain. These parts are reached and affected by sensation, movement, and breathing. The Appendix lists somatic interventions that can be done with individuals, pairs, and groups.

To illustrate the impact of societal trauma, I write of my heartfelt and intense experiences in the country of El Salvador in the next two chapters.

# Chapter Four

———•◦❀◦•———

# A PSYCHOLOGIST IN EL SALVADOR
## PART 1

Last June a visit to my daughter, Kristin, who is living and working in El Salvador, began to evolve into a professional adventure. She works for a Salvadoran NGO (NGOs are small nongovernment organizations supported by privately donated money from foreign countries, committed to work in economic development, educational development, mental health, and so on). She had met Orlando, a Salvadoran psychologist, who is a professor at the Universidad Centroamericana (UCA) and also works with the Commission for Human Rights. (The Commission for Human Rights provides medical and mental health services for people directly affected by the war.) UCA, a private university in San Salvador founded in 1965 by the Compañia de Jesus, is a project of lay persons and Jesuits established to be a critical conscience of the reality in El Salvador and to promote social change and justice. Needless to say, it was not very popular with those in power during the war. It was here in 1989 that Ignacio Martín Baró, five other Jesuit priests, their cook and her 15-year-old daughter were assassinated by the military. The soldiers dragged the bodies of the priests out into a garden, apparently as a statement. Today, a lovely rose garden blooms there, planted by the murdered woman's husband. The small room where the cook and her daughter were found has been preserved as a shrine in their memory.

Although Orlando is a traditional psychologist (psychoanalytically oriented), he took an avid interest in my work, as explained to him by Kristin. He asked that I fax him my résumé, which I did, along with a summary in Spanish of my orientation to working with trauma. Contrary to reason, I found myself saying yes when my daughter asked if I would be open to various commitments of my time while I was there.

Although I was aware of the current danger in El Salvador, I was grateful that Kristin had spared me the details until giving me travel instructions: "Don't bring any gold or other expensive-looking jewelry. Don't wear your watch. You may have to wait for a while in the airport [my plane arrived at 5:30 A.M.], because it is dangerous to drive on the highways in the dark. We will be there when you arrive, since they now have soldiers stationed along this highway to the airport."

Thirteen years of a brutal war and wanton violation of human rights has left a climate of violence in El Salvador. Such widespread trauma creates a tendency for the community to split into victims and perpetrators. The problem of impunity (those who committed the atrocities are never brought to justice) tears the social fabric to pieces, resulting in much confusion and distortion of social and moral values. Living for so many years with the life and death urgency to survive also contributes, I believe, to the destruction of the moral fiber of society and to the acting out of violence. A survival mode of existence continues long after the immediate danger has passed, resulting in a tendency toward moral chaos, corruption and hedonism. This is particularly evident among the young (delinquency and gang violence is continuously reported in the news to be out of control), but is manifested on all levels of society.

I sensed danger almost everywhere in a world in which people were always on guard. Humor often supported what seemed to be a necessary sense of denial. For instance, on one of my trips to the *campo* (countryside), we became hopelessly stuck in the mud. We were already two hours late for our meeting with a group of *campesinos* (people who live in the countryside). Kristin said that she could run the rest of the way to the community (being a marathon runner), but she wished that she had a pistol to carry with her. This became something of a joke; she was good-naturedly kidded the rest of the day about her interest in "*pistolas*." The truth was, as Kristin knew, that a young woman teacher from the community had been hacked to death in broad daylight on this very road only two weeks earlier.

One of my personal adventures included a visit with my daughter to *El Centro* (the center of the city), an experience I was not sure I would survive in one piece. At one point I looked to my right and saw a young man covered with fresh, wet blood. Even more alarming was the fact that I seemed to be more of an attraction than he was. We were warned a number of times by well-meaning people that it was too dangerous for us to be there and that we should leave immediately, an example of the fact that for every person who would hurt you there are three who would take care of you. While driving away from El Centro we became stuck in a narrow street behind a bus that would not move, no matter how hard Kristin leaned on the horn. We both began to feel alarmed, since it is not uncommon for a street to be blocked with a vehicle by people whose intention is to harm you. In such circumstances you are at their mercy, being trapped and unable to escape. Finally the bus moved, and we discovered that it had just been robbed. The doorman of the bus had gone after the thief.

Heavily armed guards were stationed outside every bank, gas station, and store. On the relatively safe upper middle-class street where my daughter, her boyfriend, (Peter, and their roommate, Raul) lived in a rented house there were three armed guards twenty-four hours a day. Everyone who lived on the street contributed money to pay them monthly. I found it curious that in this atmosphere, with my own trauma history, I felt extremely open and expansive, alert, but not fearful. I am inclined to believe that being in the presence of the Salvadoran people had much to do with this. I was deeply touched by these very warm, open, inclusive, proud, and lively people.

This description of the current atmosphere in El Salvador not only gives a backdrop for my experiences there, but also demonstrates the frightening potential for trauma to be reenacted. Those of us who work with trauma know that once an individual has been traumatized, almost certainly parts of the experience will continue to be lived out in some way. We also observe secondary trauma or trauma contamination. Those in close proximity to a traumatized person—family members or even psychotherapists—often begin to experience some of the effects of the trauma.

Intergenerational effects of trauma are well documented in the literature on child abuse and the Holocaust syndrome. Thus, when an entire population is traumatized, it is hardly surprising that there is a tendency for the trauma to be reenacted on a societal level in the form of violence. We might even hypothesize that an energetic field of violence is generated by this kind of horror.

My Argentinean friends, who lived through *la guerra sucia* (the "dirty war") in Argentina, often refer to Central and South America as *"otra planeta"* (another planet). This reminds me of one of my favorite movies, *El Hombre Mirando al Sudeste* ("Man Facing Southeast"). In this Argentinean movie the "mental patient," who becomes such a mystery for the psychiatrist, claims that he is from another planet. He tells the psychiatrist that his space ship had landed in Janin. Janin was one of the most notorious "concentration camps" where those under suspicion by the dictatorship were taken to be tortured and killed. However, my friends' way of referring to this part of the world predated the movie by many years.

In contrast to the traumatic field of violence in El Salvador, neighboring Costa Rica, where I visited next, felt peaceful and gentle. I had been to Costa Rica before and was so impressed by this little pocket of sanity in the midst of the madness surrounding it. Often I found myself wondering how this had happened. In Costa Rica I had the good fortune to fall into conversation with a man who knew a great deal about history. When I asked him this question, he told me that when the Spaniards came to Costa Rica there were almost no Indians there to rape, massacre, and enslave. The country was primarily settled by colonialists. The few Indians who lived there mostly died of disease, as did many of the colonialists—so many, in fact, that it was difficult to establish that first colony. The contrast with El Salvador supports the notion that perhaps an energetic field of trauma, setting up the urge to kill and destroy, was never established in Costa Rica.

After landing and clearing customs in El Salvador, I found that Kristin and Peter had braved the highway before dawn to meet my plane. Soon we were sitting at a roadside *pupusaria* devouring *pupusas*, the national dish of El Salvador. A ball of dough is made from rice, corn, or wheat. One can request beans or beans and cheese to be sealed inside the ball of dough. It is then flattened a bit and fried. Every table is supplied with a large jar of shredded vegetables soaked in vinegar and a tasty tomato sauce spread on top of the pupusa. They are uniquely delicious and I lived on them while I was there.

The rented house where Kristin, Peter, and Raul lived was considered luxurious by Salvadoran standards. By American standards it was badly in need of paint and repairs. The plumbing could not handle any paper being flushed down the toilets and we were without water almost every night. But it was home and I loved it, with its unkempt garden and sparse furnishings.

I caught three hours of sleep before my life began to unfold rapidly. Orlando was eager to meet me, Kristin said. That afternoon I found myself on the lovely UCA campus. Orlando received me warmly. I thoroughly enjoyed my first meeting with this highly intelligent, witty, fun-loving man. He ushered me to the office of the chairman of the psychology department, Erick. There on his desk lay my résumé and the summary in Spanish that I had faxed to my daughter. It was clear that he had studied it carefully. We made an appointment to meet again the following day.

In our second meeting we discussed at length the nature of body-oriented psychotherapy and the importance of this orientation in working with trauma. He invited me to return to El Salvador to train a group of licensed psychotherapists in a body-oriented approach to healing trauma. It was an offer I could not refuse. I know that I will not be enriched by the money involved, but by the experience. They desperately need this knowledge, and they are eager to learn about this work.

Synchronicity, which seemed to be shaping my visit to El Salvador before my arrival, continued to do so during my stay. A seminar on torture and the violation of human rights just happened to be starting four days after I arrived. A group of about thirty people from Chile, Argentina, Guatemala, Honduras, Paraguay, Uruguay, Denmark, and El Salvador were meeting for a week to share information about their work. Through Orlando, I was invited to attend the seminar. However, Orlando had also planned so many other interesting things for me during the week that I was able to attend only about half of the time.

Orlando reminded me of myself. He is very involved with his work, close to being overextended, but obviously enjoying all that he is doing. He skillfully juggles his professional life with his personal life as a single parent of two college age children. Whenever he was not able to be present for something he had planned for me, he always made sure that I was well taken care of. For instance, I arrived at a private seminar early in the morning thinking that he would be there, but he was nowhere to be seen. However, I was warmly welcomed by the woman at the desk, who clearly was expecting the American psychologist. When I entered the room of strangers sitting at tables, my feeling of being an outsider quickly turned into feeling like an insider. A lovely young woman motioned me to sit next to her. "You must be Kristin's mother," she whispered to me in Spanish; "I am Morena." I recognized her name; she was the psychologist who worked with Orlando at the Commission for Human Rights.

Within a very short time I felt quite at home. I felt so comfortable, in fact, that when I was asked by the Salvadorans at the seminar to meet with them as a group to tell them about my work, I agreed without hesitation. I found them extremely receptive and quick to grasp the material. A few in the group were already reading the Spanish translations of books by Wilhelm Reich and Alexander Lowen.

At the seminar I made a number of important connections. Among them were two Argentinean psychiatrists, who years ago helped the people in Denmark set up their center for the treatment of torture survivors. They began working with Las Madres de la Plaza de Mayo, that is, mothers of young people who were "disappeared" under the dictatorship. They continue to work in teams with torture survivors. They have written a very interesting book, *La Impunidad (Impunity)*, about how the system in Argentina engineered impunity for those who committed the atrocities and the impact of this on the society.

I also met a psychiatrist from Honduras, who truly felt like a soul brother. The orientation of his center for the treatment of torture survivors in Honduras is very much the same as the approach of our center in San Francisco. Although they don't have body-oriented psychotherapy, they work with breathing, massage, music therapy, art therapy, and herbs. He spoke eloquently of the importance of the spiritual level in healing, of the curative power of love, compassion, and caring, stressing that this is all we have in our solidarity against the violence that permeates the world today. We had a warm exchange. I confirmed my hunch that he had arrived at his holistic view through studying to be a curandero, the equivalent of a shaman or healer in Latin American countries.

I was reminded that the synchronistic world can be very small indeed when I had lunch with my daughter and her boss, Omar. He was certain that he had met me in 1991 when he was in Oakland and Berkeley for meetings with mental health professionals. I remembered a meeting some years ago at the Centro Ignacio Martín Baró in Berkeley. Many of us were crowded into the room that evening. I was surprised that he would remember me. He spent the whole afternoon with me, introducing me to the directors of several NGOs that work in the area of mental health.

In my conversations with Omar and the other directors I was impressed by their strong community orientation. They clearly understand the concept that the whole community must be healed, not just the individual. Instead of sending mental health workers or teachers into the rural communities, they carefully choose someone within the community who they feel can fill the role of mental health worker or teacher, and then train that person to work in his or her community.

I realized that I had something of great value to learn from them. Since taking over as director of the low-fee somatically oriented clinic connected with the somatics program at California Institute of Integral Studies, my intention has been to move us more toward a community orientation. I began my career working in community mental health clinics in which we really did community work. We worked with the police, the probation department, school principals, teachers, and parents. I sadly remembered that these government supported community mental health centers no longer exist in our country, the funding having been cut long ago.

Another enlightening experience was at a lunch with Kristin and her *compañeros de trabajo* (co-workers). Two of them had fled the country during the war. Jorge had gone to Costa Rica, where he worked with refugees from his own country. Gustavo lived in Denmark, where he worked very hard to raise money for the FMLN (Farabundo Marti National Liberation Front). When he returned to El Salvador after the war, he found that because of the corruption in the party some of the leaders of the FMLN had used the money for their own personal gain, rather than for social change.

Both Jorge and Gustavo spoke of their faded idealism and seemed ambivalent about expressing their current skepticism. This underlined my current belief that for the world to change, we must have a revolution in human consciousness, not just more social revolutions. Any social ideal must take into account human nature, including basic fears and basest motives; they must be faced and transcended. Revolutionary promises of change have historically ignored human psychology, to their peril.[1]

Basic understanding about trauma can be very reassuring to a survivor. I spent a good deal of time talking with Kristin's and Peter's roommate, Raul. He told me about his own war trauma and his fruitless search through the mental health system for help. Although he was on antianxiety medication, he continued to have serious panic attacks and other well-known symptoms of PTSD. I was able to share information about trauma with him, so that he had a healthier frame around his experience. Unfortunately, time constraints interfered with us working more extensively together, but we still communicate by mail.

The more I became engaged with the people, the more possibilities opened to me. I spent one afternoon with a group of psychologists and medical doctors who worked at the clinic of the

Commission for Human Rights, introducing them to a body-oriented approach to healing trauma. The experience reminded me of being with my students in California. Having limited time, I allowed their interest to guide our attention. We concentrated on the concept of character structure—the notion that everything we have lived through is structured in the body. They were fascinated with the idea that developmental issues can be approached on the physical and energetic levels as well the verbal level. We experimented with a few somatic interventions , such as those that open one's breathing and ground one's energy.

Another focus was on how persons who have been traumatized become overwhelmed with feelings related to the trauma, and how somatic interventions can help to modulate emotion. I was impressed with the stimulating questions they asked. For example, they wanted to know if I had ever worked with perpetrators? "If not, why not?"

I gave up attending the final night of the seminar on torture and the violation of human rights to give a talk at the UCA. I felt somewhat anxious about addressing this much larger and less psychologically sophisticated group. Because their knowledge about psychology in general and trauma in particular was limited, I worked hard to simplify the material. They were responsive and receptive. The questions they asked revealed their intense interest in this material.

Among my most fascinating adventures were several trips to the *campo* with doctors, psychologists, and nurses who work with the Commission for Human Rights. One of these trips was to Ahuachapan, near the Guatemalan border. This region was seriously affected by the war. The community we visited was a reconstituted community. During the war the people were on the run, living in the mountains or crossing the border to find refuge in other countries. After the war, they returned and attempted to rebuild. Each community has a leader who is trusted, and is capable of bringing the members together to pursue common goals. The Commission for Human Rights works closely with these leaders to arrange medical and psychological treatment for people directly affected by the war. NGO projects related to mental health, economic development, and educational development, such as the work my daughter is doing, are also coordinated through these community leaders.

We left early in the morning, arriving hours later at the little village near the community. After a cup of coffee, some coconut milk, and a jump start for the jeep (the motor kept dying), we headed out on the unpaved, muddy road to the community. The doctor who was driving finally pulled over to the side of the road. We climbed out of the jeep into the mud and began carrying the medical supplies up a small slope. There in a little clearing was a two-room house with a mud floor, which belonged to the leader of the community. A table was set outside the door. The doctors and nurses put on their white coats and began attending to the people waiting, who were seated on logs in front of the house.

No one seemed the least bit concerned about the likelihood that the jeep would not start when we were ready to leave, and that there were no other vehicles for miles around. This capacity to live so totally in the present was something that endeared me to the Salvadoran people.

For instance, there is far less preoccupation with time in El Salvador than what I am accustomed to in my own culture. At every appointment that I had, whether it was with the chairman of the psychology department or with the doctors and psychologists of the Commission for Human Rights, I waited from twenty minutes to an hour for the others to arrive. I found it interesting that no one apologized for being late and, probably did not even consider themselves late, suggesting a different relationship to time. The general attitude toward time seemed to be that there is always enough, whereas in my culture, the attitude is that there is never enough time, making it more difficult to sink deeply into the experience of the moment. Also, in El Sal-

vador the unexpected seemed to be accepted as a possible adventure, rather than as an impediment to a prearranged plan.

Orlando, who was unable to accompany us on this trip, had
asked me to do two consultations with members of this community. Only one of them was present. This was just as well, because it took most of the time we were there to establish trust
and then do the consultation with her. She was the wife of the
leader of the community.

She readily accompanied me to a little shack on the property,
so that we would have some privacy. Kristin was there to assist
me, should it be necessary, in understanding the *campo* dialect,
and the woman's three youngest children wandered in and out
as we talked. None of this seemed to interfere at all with her
openness. I was surprised at how easily I understood the *campo*
dialect, how responsive she was to a body-oriented approach,
and how readily I was able to come up with a treatment plan for
her extraordinarily complex case.

My task was to understand and to help her understand the
impact of what she had lived through, how this manifested in
her life now, and what might be done to help alleviate her symptoms. She became curious about how collapsed and contracted
her upper body was, which allowed only very shallow breathing.
When we worked a little with her breathing, she could sense a
slightly different experience of herself. Because there is no one
to do ongoing somatically oriented work with her, a logical and
practical suggestion was to prescribe that she get out of the
house and walk briskly, which would help her open her breathing and begin to build a more energetic charge in her body.

Walking made additional sense because another important
aspect of the treatment plan was intended to ameliorate her extreme isolation. She spent much of her time alone in the house
reexperiencing her nightmare of the past. She was quite receptive to the suggestion that she spend time with her women

friends and with the village priest and begin to share with them what was tormenting her. She would need to walk to their houses and to the village. Although this part of the treatment plan was complicated by the fact that her husband did not want her to leave the house, she asked that we talk to her husband to secure his permission for her to do this.

I further recommended that she be included in a psychotherapy group that the Commission for Human Rights was about to begin in the community. She agreed to attend without hesitation. I also consulted with the doctor about putting her on a vitamin regimen. In the course of our conversation she mentioned that her son had given her some "medicine," which helped her. She sent one of the children to fetch the empty package of pills and I discovered that the pills had been vitamins. In addition to the fact that the diet of the campesinos is limited, this woman was going through menopause, a time when many women need additional nutrients.

I left a written report and spent an hour discussing her case with a psychologist and medical doctor. In all, I spent about four to five hours to assess and initiate a treatment plan for just one woman. It is discouraging to realize that there are thousands of others in this country as deeply wounded as she.

During this interview I realized that Kristin, who was present, was becoming quite charged with emotion. As soon as we were alone she wept and wept, saying over and over again, "She has had such a hard life; she has had such a hard life." I was reminded once again of the secondary effects of trauma. Because I work with horror of this sort all the time and have lived through it myself, I have found my way over the years to being fully present for my clients without allowing myself to be traumatized by their trauma. But my daughter, in her effort to be of help in this situation, did not know what she was opening herself up to, nor did she have ways to protect herself. In discussing the experience, Kristin and I wondered whether her growing up with a traumatized mother might have made her even more sensitive to the impact of another's pain.

We all held our breath when it was time to leave the village, wondering if the jeep would start. It did. We all cheered, and soon we were eating a well-deserved meal in the neighboring village. Ironically, after lunch the jeep wouldn't start. We had to solicit a push from another vehicle to get it going. After that, the driver did not dare to turn it off again until we arrived at the Commission for Human Rights office in San Salvador.

Another day Orlando, Kristin, Morena, the young psychologist, Daniel, an Argentinian psychiatrist from the seminar, and I piled into the station wagon of the Commission for Human Rights, destined for Zacatecoluca in the departamento of La Paz (Peace).[2] We had an appointment in one of the communities there. This was a community where Kristin worked; she had made the appointment with the community leader. The jeep, which had nearly left us stranded in the *campo* the previous day, had not yet been repaired. The only other vehicle available was the station wagon, unfit, I was to learn, for negotiating the unpaved roads during the rainy season.

We were breezing along with Orlando at the wheel when Kristin noticed that we were not on the right road. Orlando was convinced there was another way to Zacatecoluca. However, we were soon quite lost and had to ask directions. Finally, we turned onto the unpaved road for which we had been searching. After a wild ride through the mud and water, Orlando chose the wrong passage, and we found ourselves hopelessly stuck in the mud. This was when Kristin offered to run the rest of the way to the community, since we were now two hours late for our appointment.

Just as Kristin was gathering herself to take off, a jeep appeared—in this area where the local folk own no vehicles. The jeep belonged to three young people working for an organization facilitating the transfer of land, an important part of the Peace Accords signed at the end of the war. They pulled us out of the mud, helped us find a safe place to leave the station wagon, stuffed us all into their jeep, and drove us to the community. They said they would find ways to occupy their time and return for us later.

Zacatecoluca is another region that was targeted by the military during the war as being sympathetic to the guerrillas. They suffered terribly as a result. Kristin had arranged to bring the Commission for Human Rights to meet with those in the community who needed medical or psychological help as a direct result of the war. When we arrived, the leader of the community and the twenty-five people he had identified were still waiting for us. Previously Kristin had attempted to organize a meeting of community members who might be interested in learning to read and write. A literacy class is offered free through her organization. But no one showed up. The same thing happened in another community, where Kristin had put in a good deal of effort. In contrast, to arrange this meeting with the Commission for Human Rights, Kristin had simply left a note with the leader of the community. The fact that not only did twenty-five people show up, but they waited for us for two and one half hours, suggests something about the reality these people are living. So many poured their hearts into the war and gained nothing, or are worse off as a result. Thus, literacy must take a back seat to dealing with the psychological and physical consequences of the war.

Juan Carlos, the leader of the community told his story. He had been picked up and tortured seven times. Each time he refused to sign anything. Yet he was far from a broken man. Although some dissociation was evident, this man exuded strength as well as softness. I could see his this as I watched him interact with his children and other community members.

Many residents were former guerrillas and torture survivors.

Juana, eighteen years old, joined the guerrillas when she was ten. (I read that about 70 percent of the guerrillas were between the ages of ten and twenty. Kristin knows her father, Esteban. He still carries in his pocket the paper that the *Fuerzas Armadas* (Armed Forces) presented to him when they arrived to take him away for two months of torture because he had been accused of subversive activity. He very much wanted to show it to us and to talk about this experience. One of his sons had also been taken away; he never returned. When asked if his whole family was involved with the guerrillas. Esteban answered, "Yes, thank God."

Orlando posed some very pertinent questions. "How is it to live side by side now with those who committed the atrocities?" Most of the former soldiers are also very poor and live in the *campo*. It was interesting to hear from these people, so devastated by the armed forces, that it is really all right. They said that many of the former soldiers feel now that they had been manipulated and brainwashed by the system. They are learning that they are really brothers. There are many "complications" in the land transfer process which they feel is not working. Sadly, they described the national police force, which was reorganized by the U.N. after the war, as slowly turning back into the repressive force it had been. Do they want another war? The answer was "yes."

I returned with an even deeper understanding of what it means to work with such seriously traumatized survivors. At times I entertain the simplistic notion that in tragedies such as this the good become even better and the bad become worse. I was so impressed with the people I met who are truly dedicated to helping their fellow human beings. At the same time, I was so horrified by the forces of evil that destroyed this once beautiful country. In addition to the traumatized population, the traumatized environment has resulted in an ecological disaster. The random violence, the prominent display of weapons and guards, and the caution in the air had a sinister feel.

I experienced something similar when I was in Tibet last year. I believe it has to do with the forces of evil pressed against the forces of goodness, love, and compassion. It is a real tribute to the resiliency of the human spirit that however powerful the repression, the forces of goodness cannot be stamped out. Tibet and El Salvador are, of course, very different, but in this respect they felt similar.

The following quote captures the essence of this truth.

*All I wanted to say is this: The misery here is quite terrible; and yet, late at night when the day has slunk away into the depths behind me, I often walk with a spring in my step along the barbed wire. And then time and again, it soars straight from my heart—I can't help it, that's just the way it is, like some elementary force—the feeling that life is glorious and magnificent, and that one day we shall be building a whole new world. Against every new outrage and every fresh horror we shall put up one more piece of love and goodness, drawing strength from within ourselves.*

ETTY HILLESUM

Westerbork Transit Camp
3 July 1943[3]

# Chapter Five

———— ❦ ————

## A PSYCHOLOGIST IN EL SALVADOR
## PART 2

It was Easter week and the airport in Costa Rica was jammed. My daughter and I were returning to El Salvador. I wanted to change some pesos back to dollars, but noticed that there was no one at the bank window. At the information desk I asked why there was no one managing the bank. I understood the response to my inquiry very well in Spanish, but in the logic of my world it made no sense. *"Están afuera en la Calle"* ("They are out in the street"). Three times I asked the same question and received the same answer. Finally, I was able to shift my mental set, and I saw that the "bank" was three men who held fistfuls of dollars on the curb outside the airport. Graciously and with no formalities that could obstruct the process, they changed money for those of us entering or leaving the country. I was shocked and impressed. Where else in the world could such large amounts of money be changing hands in a situation of such open vulnerability?

An hour later, arriving in El Salvador, I felt the difference in the energy—a jagged, unsettling, chaotic quality around me. My internal state paradoxically moved more toward calmness, being in the moment, and trusting that despite the chaos things would work out. We were met by my daughter's friend and co-worker. As we set out on the highway to San Salvador, he explained that it was no inconvenience to pick us up. He and his family had decided that the risk of being out during *Semana Santa* (Easter week, celebrated from Wednesday through Monday) was so great that it outweighed their desire to celebrate. I took in his words as I gazed out the window of the car, observing the pick-up trucks full of people, many hanging casually on the rim, cars passing wildly on the right or the left. It appeared to be a festive atmosphere flirting with danger.

The next day, which was Easter Sunday, I read in the morning paper the statistics on the number of dead and wounded from traffic accidents, drowning, rapes, and knifings. The numbers were staggering. It reminded me once again of the concept of trauma reenactment: how once an individual or a whole society has been traumatized there is a powerful tendency for parts of the traumatic experience to be re-created and lived out in some way. The professionals in my workshop in the following days found this idea made sense out of the "senseless" violence that they witness daily.

Prior to my arrival, I had arranged to accompany members of the clinic for the Commission for Human Rights on their weekly visit to one of the communities with which they work. Although I had been told about several incidents of vehicles being stopped and robbed at gunpoint in broad daylight, I found that once we were on the road, the mild anxiety I had felt disappeared.

Once again I saw how things differ in this culture. After arriving exactly on time at the clinic for the Commission for Human Rights, we left for the *campo* a full hour later, because our driver was late. The psychologist we were to pick up on the way out of town had apparently given up on us and was not at the designated site. There was no sense of frustration or worry. Such things are considered part of the process.

Our traveling team consisted of our driver, Dagoberto, a warm, sensitive, competent man who inspired a sense of security; Sara, the new director of the clinic; Marta, a medical doctor from the clinic with whom I had worked during my first visit to El Salvador; Kristin, and myself. Sara, a psychologist had returned to El Salvador four months earlier to take the position as director of the clinic. During the war she and her husband and three children had to flee when it was clear that her life was in danger because of the work she was doing. After living out the remainder of the war with her family as political refugees in Toronto, Canada, she returned to continue her dedicated work with victims of political violence. She has a grant from the United Nations almost identical to the one we have for the Center for the Survivors of Political Torture in San Francisco. She was experiencing the same anxiety we were experiencing about whether our grants would be renewed.

We were headed for a small pueblo, Conquer, surrounded by five other small communities. This pueblo and the surrounding area had been totally destroyed by military bombings and massacres during the war. It is estimated that about 80 percent of the people living in this area were tortured. Once 300 families lived in this pueblo. The area was sympathetic to and heavily populated by the guerrillas. Similar to our "scorched earth" policy in Vietnam, this pueblo and the surrounding area was razed to the ground; all the inhabitants were either killed or had to flee. Now seventy-six families have returned and are in the slow and painful process of rebuilding their community.

I was deeply touched by the symbolism of what had happened here. In front of the remnants of what once was and would again be their church, two unexploded bombs were erected as sculptures in remembrance of the punishment visited upon their village. A partially destroyed helicopter, dragged from a nearby field, had been placed next to the church, reflecting their determination to remember and acknowledge the suffering they had endured.

When we arrived at the community, we learned that the clinic was locked. The nurse, who lived somewhere in the vicinity, had the key. Unperturbed, the treatment team set up the clinic in the house of one of the community members. As Marta attended to the medical needs of the people present, Sara and I worked with one of her patients, Luis, a man in his forties, who had been imprisoned and tortured three times. Luis is married with three young children. His wife had also been tortured; she was not in treatment at that time. Sara had asked that I work with two of her patients in the community. However, after the two hours we spent with Luis, we did not have enough time.

Luis felt disoriented much of the time (he was clearly very dissociated). He felt tired and unable to sustain much activity. He found it very difficult to be in contact with other members of the community for any length of time, resulting in feeling and being quite isolated. He also had a constant headache, located in the middle front of his head. When he walked or worked in the fields his headache became worse. Sara had been helping him to reconnect to the community and to tolerate more contact. He had been able to share with her parts of his experience of torture. She had also been doing some hypnosis with him and teaching him self-hypnosis to relax. Involved and motivated in his treatment process, he was eager to work with me.

The three of us went into the bedroom of the house, separated from the rest of the house by a curtain. I asked Luis if he felt comfortable lying down on the bed. Without hesitation he said that he did. Clearly the norms we observe in the treatment frame in my own culture cannot be transferred to this situation in another culture.

Luis's body appeared to be frozen in immobility—inflexible, brittle, with no sense of fluidity, and collapsed, as well. What was apparent immediately, and is so common in survivors of extreme abuse, was that his breathing was barely perceptible. There was almost no movement in his chest or abdomen as he breathed. In addition, he constricted greatly around the exhale; it stopped in the region of his diaphragm. Because of what I had heard and observed about him in our hour-long talk, I felt it was safe to work with his breathing and energy without risking the possibility that he would flood with emotion. I had concluded this because of how dissociated he appeared to be. My thinking was confirmed when I noticed how he talked of the details of his torture experience with no affect, indicating that the emotion was very separated from the information he was imparting. In addition, I trusted my extensive experience with survivors to guide me in keeping Luis grounded in the present during this delicate venture into his self-experience.

Sara and I knew that the pain in his head could be the consequence of an actual head injury, since Luis is not able to reconstruct all that happened to him. Sara had him scheduled for a neurological exam the following week. However, my sense was that the pain was likely related to a prolonged state of shock.

It appeared to me that his energy was drawn to the center of his body and his head, and locked there in a state of immobility. This is something with which I am very familiar in my work with survivors. Luis seemed to be frozen in that state.

I began by doing some gentle exploration. When he breathed a little deeper, or I just held his head, adding energy to his system, the pain in his head increased (consistent with his report that the pain increased when he walked or worked in the fields). Initially I just held his head and asked if he could pause just a little more on the exhale. Gradually there was some expansion, some deepening of his breathing, and some movement of energy. This was slow, tedious work, yet fascinating at the same time.

At some point Luis reported feeling "*hormigas*" in his thighs and upper arms. This means "ants" in English; it is a word that my Salvadoran clients in the Center in San Francisco use when they experience energy moving into parts of their body that have been less energized. When I touched his upper arm it felt warm, compared to his lower arm, which was still cold. We continued in a similar fashion for over an hour.

By the end of the session he felt *"hormigas"* in his feet, lower arms, and hands, and indeed his lower arms and hands now felt much warmer. He reported that the pain in his head was barely there, suggesting to me that my hypothesis was correct—that the pain in his head was the result of an energetic state related to shock.

Sara sat next to us, taking notes. Our intention was for her to continue the simple work with him. She attended the following four-day workshop I taught on this type of work.

Before we left for our visit to the neighboring community, Felicita, the *dueña* of the house, fed us a generous lunch. Her husband had suffered injuries during the war that had taken his life a year earlier, leaving her with two small children. Although she struggles to survive economically, she would not allow us to leave without sharing her food with us.

Perhaps because of my background in developmental psychology and child clinical psychology, I always observe children and parents. What I saw here and in the neighboring communities was that the very young children still had the spark of life in their eyes. Older children, even those who could have been born after the end of the war, had a dull, lifeless look in their eyes. Children who were at the age of separation and individuation, who under other circumstances would flirt with strangers, moving away from their mother to explore, clung to their mothers, averted their eyes, and often hid behind their mothers. I was saddened by this and by my understanding of how the experiences of their parents and the aftermath of the war were affecting them.

During the workshop I had the opportunity to talk with some of the professionals. They told me that it is common for young children to cling to their mothers and for mothers to cling to their young children, having already lost so much—husbands and older children—to the violence of the war. Once again I was struck by the transgenerational effects of violence: how the trauma is transmitted to the next generation and on to the next.

We left Cinquera after lunch to visit one of the five surrounding communities, where Sara had a class scheduled for members of the community. When we arrived, the two *promotoras de salud mental* (mental health facilitators, who are members of the community, trained by the professionals of the clinic) were there, but other members of the community did not show up. We realized that it was *Semana Santa* (Easter, which continues through Monday); the community was still on vacation.

Although I did not have the opportunity to see Sara in action with the members of the class, I did get a sense of how she was attempting to educate them about symptoms of trauma and give them some idea of how to reduce "stress," that is, symptoms of PTSD. She had it all neatly mapped out on a makeshift flip chart. I began to fantasize about how easily basic bioenergetic exercises could be incorporated into this meeting and could even be used to help in the healing of the community in general.

In a tragedy such as this war, not only are individual identities destroyed by violence, but the identity of whole communities is obliterated. As those of us who work on a body level know, the return to who we are is through the body—the body of the individual, the body of the community. My mind continues to explore possibilities for using our body-oriented techniques, not only to restore health to the individual, but to the community as a whole. El Salvador has as one of its healing resources a very strong community orientation, which had been intentionally damaged.

Monday night I moved from my daughter's house into La Casa de Huespedes (guest house) on the campus of the Universidad Centroamericana "José Simeón Cañas." This five-bedroom, modestly but tastefully furnished house provides board and room for visiting professors and other guests. The three of us who were guests at the time were generously cared for by Mari, the housekeeper. I soon learned what the saying meant, "You will never die from hunger in La Casa de Huespedes, but from too much food." The front door of the house opened to a courtyard and then to a quiet street outside the campus. The back door opened to the campus.

This comfortable haven and easy access to the salon where I met with the group[1] was to prove very important in the demanding days ahead. This workshop was probably the most challenging thing I have ever done professionally. I was aware of deep sense of anxiety in the days before the workshop, a feeling that I never experience when approaching teaching situations. The reasons for this began to clarify during the workshop and continued to do so in the weeks that followed.

What I understand now is that, although I knew who the members of the group were, I was unable to get a sense of what being with them might be like. I have always been able to do this in any other teaching situation. I also knew that this was a very mixed group. Although the majority were psychologists, there were also six people with much less training in psychology—a doctor, two pastors, and three social workers. About half of the group were graduates of UCA (Universidad Centroamericana), the private university in San Salvador, which means that they had to come from somewhat privileged backgrounds to afford this education. Had my daughter not intervened, the whole group would have been professionals connected with UCA. This would have been easier for me, but much less interesting. Kristin wanted to make sure that people from less privileged backgrounds and those who were immersed in working with heavily traumatized communities (i.e, ex-guerrillas) were represented in the group. Thus, she met with the chairman of the psychology department, who was organizing the workshop, and planned with him who would be invited to attend.

I had asked that the group be limited to around 20 persons, since the teaching would, of course, include experiential work, and if the group were larger I would not be able to keep my finger on the pulse of what was happening. This seemed particular important with this group. Not only was I teaching body-oriented psychotherapy, which in itself generally brings much to the surface, but also I was addressing trauma, which is always very activating. In addition, I was doing this in a heavily traumatized country. Before the group started I was informed that some of the members had lost family during the war and had themselves been tortured. Thus, another concern lurking in my mind was working with this material in a society that had suffered a brutal war only four years ago.

I knew that the members had no prior knowledge of body-oriented psychotherapy. Generally, I teach groups that have had some exposure, at least to written information. My plan was to spend two days on this area and then interweave this information with that of understanding and working with trauma. I had no idea how they would receive the experiential part of the workshop. Would they think it strange? Would it be too activating? I found that this concern was totally unfounded.

Another preoccupation was vague until I spoke with Kristin and her co-worker the day after the workshop ended. We were discussing how the war had destroyed the people's sense of identity—their connection to their roots. Especially affected was the strong sense of community, historically inherent in this culture: the sense of working together to better their own situation. There is a tendency to look to "experts"—foreigners or Salvadoran professionals—to solve their problems. Yet the problem is primarily a lack of confidence, a sense of feeling disempowered.

Healing must, as always, be centered in empowering the individual and the community. I was concerned about being seen as the "expert" from abroad, who had not lived through this war, yet presumed to be able to understand and help. I found in the days to follow that I walked a narrow line, attempting to bring to them as much of my knowledge as I could, while at the same time listening to them, learning from them, and to the best of my ability fitting my knowledge with their knowledge and their needs.

What became clearer to all of us as we worked together is that these basic principles of helping one reconnect to one's body, one's roots, are applicable on the level of the community body, as well. Someone told how one NGO (nongovernment organization) had approached a literacy project with the organic process of having the members begin by building a model of their community with sticks and stones. They then began to envision what they might want to do next. Out of this organic process grew an interest in reading and writing. This is a very different approach from outsiders coming to the community and attempting to convince the members of the importance of learning to read and write, something that has not been very successful.

For the first time in my position of teacher, I shared my trauma experience with a group of students. Not only did I have serious trauma in my own past, but the worst of this was a systematic assault on my personality to destroy my memory and identity, which was an experience of torture. I added that because of this I know the healing process from the perspectives of the survivor and of the professional. This was a big step for me, but intuitively it felt necessary. By sharing this I was freed energetically to enter this four-day experience with them at a level that would otherwise not have been possible.

The first day I gave them a great deal of information. I traced the evolution of body-oriented work from Freud to Wilhelm Reich, to Alexander Lowen, John Pierrakos, and Stanley Keleman. I was attempting to give them an overview of this area, doing justice to its complexity, without getting lost in parts of it that they could not understand with so little instruction. My goal was to do this and then to focus on basic principles. This would help them begin to view the people with whom they were working through different eyes, and they could begin to work with these basic principles after the workshop.

I felt a bit of a defensive edge come up in me, which I almost never feel when I am teaching. In retrospect, I believe that there were many small challenges coming from the group, testing who I was, and who I was with them. At the end of that day, in addition to once again carefully reorganizing the material I was to teach, I found it necessary to do some work with myself on a spiritual level. I became very clear that I had important information to impart to this group, but that the most important thing was to keep my heart open, to be receptive to them, to listen carefully and to realize how much I could learn from them. It was clear that the experiential work was crucial to ground the information. It also was apparent that I needed to zero in on the basic principles of energy, breathing, grounding, restoring contact with the body, charging and discharging, resistance, and boundaries. A large agenda, but manageable, and I realized it was my job to make it manageable.

The second day trust began to build in the group, but it never reached the level that we usually expect in a four-day experience. This made absolute sense to me in a society where just four years before, saying the wrong thing in the wrong place could cost you your life. Even knowing this, I was not prepared for how the work remained on the surface. My work with individuals never deepened beyond just staying with the energy, with breathing and general issues such as letting down and surrender. The problem was that this superficiality made it more difficult to get across to them how this approach actually is psychotherapy, meaning that people work very deep issues, facilitated by the inclusion of the physical and energetic levels of experience.

Gradually, they understood more and more how this process worked. The work in dyads and triads helped, as people felt able to be more open in these smaller groups. During the breaks I was able to get an idea of how much was being opened up but not spoken in the group. The members would want to talk with me personally about their experiences, apparently trusting me with this, but not the group. Later I heard that one of the members, a professor at UCA, had wanted to present a case, but declined because he felt it was "not safe" to do so. This went on, even though the general climate of the group in other ways felt just like that of any other group I have ever taught. The members worked sincerely and deeply on themselves in the experiential group work. However, when they shared, it was clear that they shared only the surface level of what they had experienced.

On the third day I introduced the field of trauma and began to weave what we had worked with into this theory. My general outline of what to cover included the history of this field of knowledge, from the studies of hysteria by Freud and his colleagues to the present. I outlined the distinction that I make between developmental trauma and shock trauma. Other important areas I wanted to cover were memory and trauma, dissociation, the psychobiology of trauma, trauma reenactment, and some basic principles in the treatment of trauma. I taught and they worked experientially with some very simple, basic somatic interventions that I find useful and safe in working with trauma.

According to trauma reenactment theory, once someone is traumatized, parts of the experience are almost sure to be lived out in some way. This theory explained for them so much of what they observed in individuals with whom they worked and in the society as a whole. We discussed how the process in a traumatized society parallels that in a traumatized individual: denial, dissociation, the destruction of identity, the lack of integration of the traumatic experience, the problem of impunity and its effects, and the reenactment of trauma.[2]

Enrique, a psychologist with an NGO that works with communities of ex-guerrillas, expressed his concern about the extent of denial and dissociation on a societal level. He said that the past ten years are referred to as "the lost decade," meaning that people are behaving and talking as though the war never happened. Others related what was happening in their country to what had happened in Germany, Argentina, and Chile. Enrique knows someone who lives right next to the home of the murderers of his family. This is not at all uncommon—that the victims and the perpetrators live side by side. Another woman he knows has one son who was a guerrilla and one who was a soldier. Many expressed their concern about the problem of impunity— that there is still no recognition of the crimes against humanity and no apology from the government for what happened.

Enrique also related a personal experience about how the effects of trauma manifest on a societal level. In a community of ex-guerrillas where he is working to establish a clinic, he was waiting for a ride in the morning. An ex-guerrilla attacked him. Five of his attacker's friends were waiting nearby. In addition to losing all of his belongings, Enrique was badly beaten. No one in the community came to his aid, even after the attackers had left. Enrique's explanation was that they are still living with too much fear. Fortunately, some people who were working with another organization came along and helped him.

There was much discussion about the random violence in the society as a whole, in particular the problem of delinquency. Research in the U.S. shows that adolescents act out rather than experience the other symptoms of PTSD, such as anxiety and depression. Thus, it is hardly surprising that it is this age group that is reenacting the violence on a large scale. Just before my visit to El Salvador, a law was enacted allowing the police to pick up any juvenile who is not working or in school and take him or her to jail, without any judicial process. This is a radical attempt to deal with the delinquency that is becoming increasingly out of control. However, it is an alarming return to the past, when the police were the law. I was told that the judges are organizing to protest the new law.

Alfonso, a pastor with a long history of working with the poor and victims of violence, asked the group what they felt they could do as professionals to help heal the trauma from the war. He was especially interested about healing on the level of the community. This is a very important resource in this culture, which has a long history of community organization and activity. We all agreed that one obvious need was to help the people keep their memories of the war alive by talking about what had happened and how it is affecting them now; to acknowledge this and to keep acknowledging it. One of the things I found to be true in my two visits to El Salvador is that the people really want to talk about what happened. I was a total stranger from a foreign land, but when they sense my openness to listening, they will talk and talk.

Sara, the director of the clinic for the Commission for Human Rights, spoke of her efforts to organize the communities in which she works around the healing process. Heidi, the one American in the group and also a pastor, told the story of a woman who had been dreadfully tortured. When she returned to her community, they took it upon themselves to help her heal. She was never left alone; someone was with her at all times. The woman carried a great deal of guilt. Because she had given names under torture, she felt she was responsible for everyone else who had been tortured. In a ritual with the community, she asked the pardon of all those she believed she had endangered. In this process it became clear to her that the others did not see her as responsible for their suffering, as she had imagined.

We spoke of the importance of ritual in the healing process. Enrique said that he knows people who are still waiting, after fifteen years, for their sons or daughters or other family members to reappear. Thus, they are never able to live through the grieving process. Many of these professionals are helping those who have lost family members to search for their graves and to perform some kind of ritual to "bury" their lost loved ones.

Jorge, another psychologist, spoke of the responsibility he and other psychologists feel for the process of healing, and how it is impossible to take on all of this. I learned that the professionals felt very connected with each other in their work during the war, but now feel very isolated. Apparently this network of connection among professionals was also seriously disrupted—I am sure largely due to the fact that it was potentially dangerous to be doing this work with victims of political violence. I pointed out that even in a culture such as my own, where there is no physical danger inherent in working with victims of abuse, it is always political, in the sense that it is not well received. Society wants to deny the truth. To do this work, wherever one does it, is to expose the truth.

In connection with this, we addressed the importance of taking care of oneself when doing this work. I emphasized that probably the most important thing is not to do this work without support from colleagues. I felt concerned for these professionals who seemed to be working under conditions that afford them little support and contact with each other. At the end of the workshop, we spent some time organizing a support group and network.

By the end of the fourth day, I felt the group had evolved. We were all feeling very satisfied and grateful for what we had experienced together. They gave me some generous feedback about my presence, how I embody what I teach, and how I do not evoke resistance or defensiveness from the group.

I was intrigued by several of Orlando's ideas. He was interested in my going to Colombia to teach there. He lived in Colombia for six years, where he worked with victims of political violence. Now he realized that they were working "blind," with no knowledge of what they were doing. In Costa Rica, where they were doing a great deal of work with torture survivors, Orlando meets once a year with a group of professionals from a number of different Central American countries. He expressed an interest in my meeting with this group.

One evening after the workshop my daughter related a touching story, reminding me that the robberies and other violent acting out, although accentuated by trauma reenactment, are also part of a bleak economic reality. The driver for Kristin's NGO told her the following story. He and two other people who work for the organization were stopped on their way to a community in the area of Cinquera, where we had traveled the day before the workshop began. The road was blocked; the men who stopped them were heavily armed and wore ski masks. But the driver and his co-workers knew they were from the community in which they worked. As the driver continued with the story, he began to weep. The robbers took all his money (his whole paycheck for the month) which was in cash. One of the other men pleaded with the robbers not to take his wedding ring because of its sentimental value. Then the robbers told them that they did not really want to rob them, but felt they had no choice. They said they could not get what the government had promised them, not even seed or fertilizer. Feeding themselves and their families was becoming impossible. Then they began to negotiate how much they would take from them. They returned half of the driver's money to him, and they did not take the wedding ring. Through their work with the campesinos, these men who work with the NGO know this hard economic reality. Thus, they came away from this experience more deeply moved emotionally than resentful or angry.

For several weeks after my return home, I felt a deep sense of grief. It seemed to be a mixture of grief for what the people of El Salvador had lost, for what I had lost so many years ago through being severely abused, and also for the loss of being immersed in the experience of their society, with which I seem to identify at a very deep level. Gradually I began to understand why I feel so comfortable emotionally among the Salvadorans. Even when physically uncomfortable or in danger, I feel a profound sense of being at home when I am there. Interestingly, while I love the beauty, safety, and comfort of Costa Rica, I do not experience there the same deep sense of emotional comfort. I feel more as I do in my own country. Thus, returning to my geographical home meant losing this sense of connection to others through my own violent past at some profound level of human experience. In addition to my desire to share my knowledge with people deeply in need of it and to have a rich learning experience for myself, there seems also to be a powerful energetic resonance that draws me to this part of the world.

# Chapter Six

———— ❧ ————

## COLLEEN'S STORY:
## A SURVIVOR OF A NEAR FATAL ACCIDENT

"I am terrified that I have brain damage, "stated Colleen, after describing for me a long list of symptoms she was experiencing.

"What you are describing are symptoms of posttraumatic stress disorder, not brain damage," I responded confidently, somewhat going out on a limb.

Colleen had just told me that she had experienced a serious bicycle accident involving a critical head injury sixteen months prior to our meeting. She described herself as feeling highly anxious and hypervigilant; she felt unsafe and as though she could not protect herself. At times she felt very helpless. Sometimes she was unable to think clearly. She had difficulty relaxing and problems sleeping; she felt very uncomfortable driving, because she had difficulty orienting her head from side to side. She did not feel "in" her experience as she had before the traumatic incident. She felt a sense of having no future. Her energy was low. In the three months following the bike accident, she had two car accidents, one of which landed her in the hospital once again. I was reminded of the powerful tendency for trauma to be reenacted. Later in her treatment Colleen would tell me about nine previous accidents and illnesses that she had experienced, including a tonsillectomy at age four.

When Colleen told me that she was going skiing the following weekend, I educated her about trauma and reenactment and held my breath. I explained how there was a strong pull for traumatic incidents to be reenacted. I surmised that her defensive and orienting responses had been knocked out in her bicycle accident, which contributed to the following car accidents and the fact that she felt so unsafe when driving. I cautioned her to stay present and grounded on the slopes, to take it easy and not to push herself (as she is so inclined to do). She did, in fact, have a successful and enjoyable skiing trip. The experience furnished us with immediate material for beginning to build a healing vortex. The memory of the strength she felt in her legs while skiing proved to be an important resource as we began treatment.

I had seen Colleen in psychotherapy for a year three and a half years earlier. She was then a student in a psychology program and needed to satisfy the psychotherapy requirement. She was then forty-three years old, a bright and very accomplished professional woman. We worked on her developmental issues during this year. She worked hard and accomplished a great deal in a short period of time.

When she returned in October of 1997, she had completed her schooling and internship and had gotten married. She had a demanding job as a professor and psychotherapist. Her life appeared to be working extremely well, except that it was contaminated by the remnants of the traumatic bicycle accident.

Colleen and I worked together in weekly one and a half hour sessions for a year and eight months. There were some long breaks when one of us was out of town.

It is important when working with head injuries to make sure the process goes at a very slow pace, because so much energy is compacted and stored in the nervous system at the moment of impact. In trauma involving high impact, even more energy is compressed in the nervous system than in other forms of trauma (Levine, 1997). The energy must be carefully titrated so that the discharge takes place extremely slowly. While Colleen was seated in a chair, there was a continuous trembling through her legs and feet; it was the intense energy discharging as we worked. Our focus was the traumatic bicycle accident. Her developmental issues were engaged at times, but the working through of the bike accident remained in the foreground.

Colleen's nervous system was very well set up to do this work. She was basically healthy, with many resources, and it was easy to establish a healing vortex (a reservoir of positive and healing experience) at the outset. She had many positive memories, including the important ones of skiing and experiencing the strength in her legs. She had many people in her life, especially in her work, who provide her with positive feedback about herself and her work. And she was in a very good marriage, which furnished her with much nourishment and support.

From the outset Colleen was able to weave between the trauma vortex and the healing vortex on her own with little intervention from me. While working in the trauma vortex she would often state that she had been distracted. I would ask her where she had gone. Invariably she had moved to a memory, or image, or a sensation that was part of the healing vortex. For instance, we might have been deeply involved in processing some piece of the accident, and in an instant she would be thinking about something that happened at work, generally involving some kind of positive input. I would encourage her to talk about the incident and to notice what she was feeling in her body as she did so. Or she might begin seeing oriental images or images of Italian ceilings, which were very beautiful and produced positive, soft feeling in her body.

When we began treatment Colleen remembered almost nothing of the accident. She had memories of the time before the accident and memories of being in the hospital and at home

afterward. Thus, much of our work involved reassociating dissociated fragments of the experience. By the time we had completed her work, Colleen remembered every detail of what had
happened. At the same time, we were attempting to uncouple
overcoupled elements of the incident. It was the overcoupling of
parts of the experience that resulted in her hyperarousal and in
her feeling flooded and overwhelmed with panic, terror, and
grief.

Her work proceeded from the periphery of the incident (what
she remembered before and after the shock core) to the intensity of the heart of the experience (being thrown from the bike and
the impact with the ground). This progression from the periphery of the experience winding slowly into the core is described by
Levine (1997) as an important, natural process when working
through traumatic material. Colleen's work progressed in this
way with little or no direction from me, and also reflected an interesting linear progression. Driving to my office, deeply immersed in the work, Colleen would feel very much the same as
she had felt at the end of the previous session. It was as though
her internal experience picked right up where we had left off the
week before. Most of the material we worked with was implicit
memory or Colleen's somatosensory experience. At times she
brought in declarative, narrative memories, but the essence of
the working through was putting implicit memory into longterm
declarative memory.

During an initial session Colleen experienced herself as she
did the day of the accident. Her body felt extremely heavy and
tired. She felt herself pedaling her bike, despite her fatigue, and
could see the road and the vegetation passing by. I encouraged
her just to be in this experience. The energy moving through her
legs intensified, and she reported feeling fear. I asked where in
her body she felt the fear. She said she felt fluttery sensations in
her upper chest. As she focused on these sensations, she shifted
on her own to the healing vortex. "I hear the clocks ticking," she

said, bringing herself into the present, "and I hear bells ringing outside." She began to talk about an amusing incident at work, one that had brought her some satisfaction, increasing her immersion in the healing vortex.

She shifted back to the trauma vortex, but this time she was in the aftermath of the accident. The lower back part of her head, where she had the hematoma was throbbing with pain. "I feel sick; I think I threw up a lot in the hospital. I see bright lights; there are lots of people around." She remembered, through her experience and from information given to her by her husband and other people, a good deal of what happened to her after the accident in the hospital. She felt the intensity of the pain and the nausea, and when she had had enough, she once again shifted to the healing vortex, this time seeing a variety of roofs. "It is as if the roofs can protect my head," she said dreamily.

At this stage Colleen also processed much of what she experienced after returning home from the hospital. She remembered sitting motionless on the sofa for hours, unable to do anything. She recalled inappropriate things that well-meaning people had said to her. With a sense of humor, she told several incidents reflecting her inability to process cognitively. Her attitude indicated a certain amount of healing had already taken place, because Colleen was able to amuse herself with these incidents, rather than scare herself. On one occasion she had decided to clean the cupboards in the kitchen. She took everything out of all the cupboards, only to discover that she was totally unable to think about how to organize them and put them back. There she was when her husband came home, sitting baffled in the dismantled kitchen. Another time she tried to make sandwiches for a picnic. She found she couldn't figure out how the sandwiches fit together after partially making them. Experiences such as these initially frightened Colleen, but within a short time after beginning our work she relaxed, seeing them as temporary impairments of her cognitive ability. She could observe that such experiences never occurred in her present life and that the symptoms she had been suffering with when she began treatment with me were slowly beginning to improve.

For about the first three months of treatment our work brought us gradually to the core of the traumatic accident. Colleen found herself sitting in the chair curled up into the position she had assumed upon impact with the ground. Her body would wind its way into this position and she would say, "The pull to go here is so strong; it is magnetic." I heard this as reflecting the strength of the pull to the trauma vortex, the magnetic attraction to repeat parts of the traumatic experience. We later discovered that Colleen had actually bounced upon impact and ended up in another pose. Her husband was with her during the accident and his report of what he witnessed confirmed her experience.

Colleen also experienced many more details of the immediate aftermath of the accident. She felt herself being strapped to a stretcher and experienced irritation at having an oxygen mask placed over her face. She heard the whirring of the helicopter that was to lift her from the scene of the accident. Sometimes she experienced herself on the stretcher and in the helicopter, and at other times she saw herself and the scene of the accident from above, very far up in the sky. During this period the tonsillectomy she had at age four would weave itself into the processing of the accident. "My throat feels so sore," Colleen would complain. "I see a bright light. Now I see the operating table and the doctor from above," she stated in a somewhat distraught voice. "I can't move." She seemed to go in and out of her body, releasing a great deal of energy as she did so. At this point I intervened, directing her to the healing vortex by asking her if she could bring to mind the memory of herself skiing. She immediately relaxed, commented on the strength she felt in her legs, and continued to discharge energy through her legs and feet.

About four months into treatment Colleen came to several

sessions feeling very emotionally charged, fearful, and angry. She said she felt afraid that she would die, or that she would "go too fast." I began by having her keep her eyes open so that she could stay connected to the present. As she looked around, she felt the pull to the trauma vortex. She felt her blood begin to pulsate and her heart to pound, and she saw images of the trail and the ground coming up at her. She had been skiing again the prior weekend. She began talking about skiing; I encouraged her. Soon she was standing and making skiing movements, feeling the strength in her legs. She would make a skiing turn and say, "and I can stop; and I can stop."

"Yes, you can stop," I repeated back to her. One of the horrors that Colleen had gotten in touch with was the realization at the moment she flew from the bike and again after she was on the ground that she could not stop what was happening; that there was nothing she could do to control the terrible thing she was experiencing. Her memory of skiing brought back the feeling that she could stop, that she had some control over what happened to her.

After this experience in the healing vortex, I directed Colleen to touch the edges of the sensations and images of the trauma vortex and then come back into the present and the healing vortex. Through this process I was attempting to help her feel more in charge of her experience, to slow her process down, and to help her begin to integrate pieces of the core of the shock experience. She felt strength in her arms and legs and power in her body. She was aware of feeling anger and saying, "I don't want you to do that," speaking to those who were charged with "doing things to her" after the accident. Her head was moving slightly from side to side, indicating that her orienting responses were being restored. In fact, after several sessions in which her head movement was quite pronounced, she reported that she felt much more safe and sure of herself while driving. Her arms also began to make slight pushing movements, indicating that her defensive responses were being activated. One of the things that Colleen expressed over and over again during her work was how impotent her arms and hands were during the accident. They felt numb and glued to the handlebars of her bike as she was thrown to the ground.

The following session Colleen arrived feeling activated and fearful. She again said that she feared she would die and had no idea what this meant. I began by having her focus on her fear sensations, which she felt primarily in her upper chest. She became more calm as she focused on them and discharged a large amount of energy through her legs.

Around this time Colleen began to realize just how serious this accident was. A very important defense for trauma survivors is denial, and Colleen had been in a state of denial. Her assimilation of the seriousness of the incident continued for well over another year; it was as though she could only integrate the reality of her injury very slowly. As Colleen calmed down, she saw healing images, like looking down from the sky and seeing geometric designs and beautiful architecture.

In one remarkable session, she began to feel drugged and she slumped slightly in her chair. What was to follow left both Colleen and me in awe. Initially, it frightened her. But later her experience became an important part of her healing vortex.

Colleen's body drew itself into the curled-up fetal position— the final resting position after she had bounced on the pavement. Her breathing was labored. She felt tremendous pain in her head and neck. She said, "I feel as though I could disappear." She pulled back slightly and said that she felt fear. Then her eyes became transfixed. Her head moved forward and to the right. "It's a tunnel," she said. "I don't feel my body; it feels so peaceful; there is no pain. The light; it is so bright." Her eyes squinted. "I want to go in; I want to go into the tunnel, to the light."

Suddenly she pulled back. She experienced the throbbing in her head and neck. Her breathing was labored. "This feels terrible," she said. "It is so peaceful there; I wanted to keep going, but I was afraid I wouldn't come back. What is going on? I don't understand what is happening."

Colleen had read nothing about near-death experiences. I had not only read about near-death experiences, but had worked with other clients who had had such experiences. I encouraged her to just stay with her experience; I told her that what was happening was quite exceptional, and that things would gradually become clearer. She went back to her labored breathing and the pain she was experiencing in her body.

"It is such a relief; it is as though I can leave my body and feel nothing but peace. Now it looks like a cave. "There is so much light; the light looks bluish now. Something feels familiar; it is as though there is someone there who feels familiar." She then came back into her body and was aware of the throbbing of her head, the pain in her neck, and her heavy breathing.

"I must have left my body; I must have died," Colleen stated, her eyes wide with fear.

"It would appear so," I responded. We were both in tears after this initial exposure to her near-death experience. I explained to Colleen that she might feel frightened by this knowledge now, but that eventually she would probably come to see this experience as a gift. that would greatly enrich her life.

We revisited this episode of Colleen losing all contact with her body, being drawn to a light and a tunnel or cave, feeling magnetically drawn in and not wanting to come back. During several of the experiences she was told that she must return to her body when she felt so drawn to the light that it felt almost impossible to return.

Colleen soon lost her fear and misgivings of the experience and began to trust that she had most likely left her body just after the final impact, during the half-hour before any medical attention arrived. As we continued to work with the near-death experience and the details of the shock core, we began to suspect that she might have left her body twice and come back, once just after the final impact and again just before being strapped to the stretcher and put into the helicopter. Soon her near-death experience became part of her healing vortex, a place that Colleen could visit to gain respite from the grueling task of working through the core of the near-fatal accident.

As she integrated more details of the traumatic incident, especially the near-death experience and the knowledge of how critical the incident was, Colleen's grieving deepened. It continued for almost a year. The depth of her grief was interesting, considering that she had made a complete recovery from the accident.

After six months of treatment, dramatic relief of her symptoms was obvious. Colleen could drive her car and feel safe and relaxed. She felt much less helpless. She felt more confident and less overwhelmed in her work. She no longer worried about having brain damage. She felt more spontaneity, less constriction, and more expansive. "I feel more myself, as I was before the accident. My sex life is better and I laugh more. I can even let down and take naps at times." Yet she still did not feel as she had prior to the accident, and her relief from symptoms was not stable. Her process seemed to have a life of its own. I trusted her unconscious mind to guide us toward more complete healing.

Colleen had recovered a good deal of her memory of the accident and its aftermath. First emerging as implicit memory or somatosensory experience, much of what had happened was now in her long-term, narrative memory. When relating long-term, declarative memory of the incident, Colleen would speak in the past tense, telling a story of what had happened.

"I remember pedaling up the hills on the way to Inspiration Point. I felt very tired, but was determined to prove that I could do the ride anyway. We were on the trail and I was behind Al. My legs felt sluggish and my breathing was heavy. I decided that I was going to pass him. I speeded up. My hands feel numb"—she switched to the present tense and began to report her so-matosensory experience, indicating that this part of her experi-ence was still encoded in implicit memory only—"my heart is pounding; I see the pavement going by. I am passing Al and I see that the trail turns and goes uphill. I feel my blood coursing and pulsating, like this," and she made a rhythm with her hand on her leg. "My breath is so high in my throat." Her eyes looked wide with fear. I knew I must slow her down or she would expe-rience too much intensity and terror.

"Just notice your breath in your throat. Follow it up and then down again; just focus on that one little piece." She did as I sug-gested, and her body discharged a great deal of energy down through her legs and feet. She calmed down and became en-grossed in the sensations of her breath in her throat. She then said that she felt distracted. I asked where she was.

"I see Italian ceilings, beautiful ones, like I saw on a trip to Europe. Now I see castles." Her body calmed and her breathing became normal. She had relieved herself by switching to the healing vortex. I encouraged her to explore her images here, and as she did she became amused, having learned to trust this pen-dulum effect of swinging between the two vortices.

She then found herself again in the near-death experience.

"I am going in headfirst," she said. "There is so much white mist, and the center is dark. There is no pain; it is so peaceful, so quiet. Someone else is making the decision; someone outside of myself is telling me to go back. I wonder who?" She then ex-perienced herself lying on the pavement; she saw the weeds; she felt the pain in her head and neck. Her breathing was heavy. "I am being lifted; I feel held down; I don't like it. Al told me that I told the medics not to strap me down. Am I in the helicopter? I see the back of a man's head; is it the pilot?"

For a time our work proceeded in this fashion, weaving between the trauma vortex and the healing vortex as we wound more deeply into the core of the accident. For quite a long time we worked on the parts of the event just before the shock core (leaving the bike and flying through the air) and the segments of the experience after impact with the pavement. This had to be done slowly because the intensity of the energy was enormous, and the release of energy had to be carefully titrated. It was important to keep Colleen's level of fear to a minimum. I modulated this carefully by getting detailed reports from her about how she was experiencing herself between sessions. If she reported that she had felt agitated or anxious or that she had had difficulty letting down or sleeping, I would back off from working with the details of the accident and work with her breathing and with grounding. I would encourage her to talk about positive experiences in her life and to fully experience herself as she did so.

Next we worked through the very core of this terrible accident, how Colleen was able to remember explicitly all the details of what happened when she lost control of her bike and flew through the air, and how she gradually and painstakingly slowly put this into declarative, long-term memory.

"I felt so tired and heavy driving up here," reported Colleen at the beginning of her session.

"Let's just start with this," I responded. "Just let yourself go into the tiredness."

"I am on my bike; I am so tired that I can hardly keep pedaling," she said. Colleen was feeling very tired that day, and she became more fatigued during the long ride. She denied her exhaustion and just kept pushing herself to keep going and to keep up with her husband. This was important information about herself that worked against her that particular day.

" I am going to pass Al; I see the trail up ahead and how it turns. I speed up. My heart is pumping so hard. My hands—they are numb. I turn and my weight shifts." Her body shifted and pulled upward.

I said, "There, notice that movement." She made the movement again.

"Oh, that is what happened; that is how I lost control; my weight shifted this way instead of like this." She made the movement again. "That is how I lost control and flew off the bike." She began to rise out of the chair, but she was gripped with fear. She felt immobilized. "I am going to disappear," she gasped. I asked her to open her eyes, and I took her hands in an effort to bring her quickly back to the present.

Energy discharged through her legs. I saw that she wanted to put pressure on her legs, and I asked her to stand and bend her knees. She felt strength in her legs and began to calm down as she held onto my hands.

"I now see what happened," she stated, beginning to put the experience into declarative memory. "I was so tired and instead of slowing down, I speeded up and passed Al. I couldn't use my hands; they were numb. I tried to turn the bike at the end of the trail where it went up, but was unable to do so. My weight shifted the wrong way. I lost my balance." She was sitting down again.

"My feet," she said as she jerked each one. "I am trying to get them out of the clips; I can't do it; they are stuck. I must not have been able to get them undone from the clips," she said, moving this information into her long-term memory.

Her body now curled into her position on the ground after the impact. "This is how I landed in the final position," she said. "My head hurt so much and I felt so sick. I can remember the helicopter coming. I was so angry when they strapped me down. They asked me questions. I couldn't answer them," she said, now amused by something that not so long ago had frightened her.

This aftermath of the accident was also now in long-term memory. She was able to relate the details with little or no charge or emotion.

"I see the blue light," she sighed, suddenly shifting. "Now it is bright white light. There is an eye; it is huge. I am in the near-death experience. It is so peaceful, so quiet." Here she was drawing on the near-death experience as part of the healing vortex. She sat quietly for a time, taking in the profound nature of what she was perceiving. Soon she looked at me and told me she felt much calmer.

I asked her to sit on a large gymnastic ball and to bounce gently as we talked. In this way Colleen was able to ground herself at the end of sessions. We generally had to spend about ten minutes or more grounding her in the present, making sure that she was feeling stable and fully connected to herself and the present before she left my office.

"It is getting clearer to me what happened," she said. "It is so terrifying; that part where I fly off the bike; I feel like I am going to be annihilated." This very core of the trauma was still not worked through. The intensity of the energy stored here and the accompanying terror was making it difficult for us to move through this portion of the event. We had worked with material on both sides of the shock core. Most of the remainder of the accident was now in long-term, declarative memory.

At the very core of the shock experience Colleen experienced herself on her bike, her blood coursing through her and her breath being inhaled in short steps as she began to feel herself lift off the bike to fly through the air. We worked with this part very slowly and in pieces. I would ask her to focus on the three short inhalations and then come back down into exhalations—going back and forth so that she could begin to feel that she had some control over her body. This was also an attempt to uncouple the overcoupled sensations.

I also asked her to focus on the coursing of the blood and then to center her attention once again on her breath. I suggested she make the lifting motion just a little and then come back to settling on the bike (in her chair). As we worked in this way, a great deal of energy was discharged through her legs and in small movements in her body. Her terror was less, but still too intense for us to move through the experience. She would switch on her own to the healing vortex, or I would direct her there. She would have images of gardening, feeling her hands in the dirt. She felt the warmth of her cat sleeping next to her in her bed.

The images associated with the healing vortex became more archetypal as we worked more deeply into the shock core. According to Levine (1997), the increase in archetypal images as one approaches the shock core is typical in working through shock trauma material. For instance, Colleen saw images of Asian gods and goddesses. I often observed that her hands were in the position of *mudras* (symbolic hand gestures).

During one session, as we were working with the shock core, I could see that Colleen was not breathing down into her viscera at all. I mentioned this, and she responded, "Yes, this is the part that is still damaged," as she placed her hand on her belly.

I realized that it was essential to do some hands-on work and asked Colleen if she was open to this. Colleen was a traditional psychotherapist, and I realized that I had avoided using touch with her, probably to the detriment of the work. But she was very open to this suggestion.

I asked her to lie on the couch. I suspected that direct touch to her diaphragm or the area of her viscera would be too activating for her. When I tried this, my hypothesis was confirmed.

I then proceeded to work to open the four diaphragms (Levine; personal communication). I gently placed my hands on either side of her head and waited until I felt the tissue expand. For me, this experience is somewhat like feeling the tissue coming out to meet my hands. I then moved my hands to the outside of her arms and waited for the same phenomenon to occur. This was a slow process, but one that was clearly very calming for Colleen. I then placed my hands on the periphery of her regular diaphragm and waited again. Her breath was lengthening and slowly moving more deeply into her abdominal area. Finally, I put my hands on either side of her pelvis, and at this point her breath elongated down into her viscera. I noticed a twitching in her toes, and her feet moved in a slight rolling motion. This indicated to me that the wave of energy that moves through the body, which is always so drastically disturbed in trauma, was in the process of being restored.

I worked in this fashion with Colleen for almost an hour and a half. When we finished, she sat up and distinctly felt a sense of the wave of energy and a strong sense of hope. She felt "high" when she left. At the beginning of the next session, she reported that she had felt light and hopeful all week.

When Colleen returned for the following session, she told me that she had felt some hyperarousal when driving to the session. As she sat in the chair, I observed that her breathing tended to be high in her chest and throat on the inhalation and that it was not descending completely into her viscera on the exhalation. I decided that another hands-on session of resourcing was in order before continuing the work in the shock core. Colleen agreed.

Again I asked her to lie on the couch and worked with my hands on the periphery of her body, starting with her head. After about an hour we once again observed the movement in her feet, indicating that the wavelike motion of energy was moving through her body. When she sat up, she said she felt very calm and peaceful.

During the following session, Colleen stated that while driving to the session she had felt a little of the hyperaroused state that we had come to recognize as part of the shock core, but she had not felt the terror that generally was associated with it. This suggested that the terror was beginning to uncouple from the sensations that made up the shock core. I could see that, although her breath was high in her chest on the inhale, there was movement in her viscera when she exhaled. I began with some resourcing by suggesting she bring her attention to her legs. "They feel strong and solid," she stated. "I am remembering my cat curled up next to me; I feel her warmth."

"Good." I responded. "Just take time to take that in."

"Now I see the blue light; then the white light. I feel so peaceful. I don't know when I have ever felt so peaceful. Maybe that is the message of the near-death experience—to find peace in this life."

She then found herself in the trauma vortex. "I feel my blood —it is moving so fast. My breath—it is high; it is going boom, boom, boom. My heart is pounding." She was aware of the sensations, but she was not experiencing the terror as she had on previous occasions.

"Focus on your heart, then on your breath, then back on your heart," I instructed her, still working to help her uncouple the overcoupled sensations. As she did this everything slowed down. Her breathing calmed, her heart beat more slowly, and the blood did not seem to be coursing so fast through her body. She then was able to bring in another dissociated piece of the traumatic event.

"I am leaving the bike," she said, rising up in her chair. "I feel so surprised and know I can't stop myself. I feel paralyzed; I can't feel my body." She experienced herself flying through the air; then her head hit the ground, and she sensed her brain bouncing to the front of her head.

"I feel so much relief; I have all the pieces," she said. "I see an old Oriental man with a long beard; there is an ornate building."

She described the architecture in detail. Her hands were in the form of a mudra. She felt calm and peaceful as she touched the healing vortex.

I suggested that we go through this part of the accident once again. "I was passing Al when I saw how the road turned up ahead, " she began. As we processed the core of the accident several more times, she related more and more of the event in the past tense, indicating that it had been put into long-term, declarative memory.

During the following session Colleen was able to tell the details of the whole traumatic accident from beginning to end. She told it in the past tense, with no emotional charge, which amazed her. She remained in the present as she narrated the whole incident.

Her grieving was now very light. She felt sadness about the accident, and also about the fact that it was time to terminate her therapy. She felt mildly despairing that I was the only person to whom she could relate her near-death experience. She was still integrating her near-death experience as we ended her therapy, knowing that it was going to have an important impact on the way she lived the remainder of her life.

When we ended, her symptoms were virtually nonexistent. She was reasonably free from hyperarousal and from feeling overwhelmed. Her anxiety level was normal. She could orient herself easily and drive comfortably. She could relax and take naps. She felt "in" her experience, felt spontaneous, and noticed that her sense of humor had returned.

Colleen knew that the accident had transformed her forever in unknown ways. She had completed her grieving over the accident and was ready to embark on her life from a new and unknown place within her.

# Chapter Seven

──── ⋅⟨◉⟩⋅ ────

# EDITH'S STORY: A SURVIVOR OF POLITICAL TORTURE

*Anyone who has been tortured remains tortured . . .*
*Anyone who has suffered torture never again will be*
*able to be at ease in the world, the abomination of the*
*annihilation is never extinguished.*
*Faith in humanity, already cracked by the first slap in the*
*face, then demolished by torture, is never acquired again.*

JEAN AMÉRY[1]
*THE TORTURE EXPERIENCE*

Torture survivors have come face to face with the evil that is possible in human interaction. They have experienced complete loss of control over their own lives, their own bodies. Systematic breaking down of their humanity, their individuality, leaves them questioning their capacity to function in the world and even their willingness to remain in a world so destructive and unjust.

The United Nations Declaration defines political torture as:

*Any act by which severe pain or suffering, whether physical or mental, is intentionally inflicted on a person for such*

*purposes as obtaining from him or a third person informa-*
*tion or confession, punishing him for an act he has com-*
*mitted or is suspected of having committed, or intimidating*
*him or a third person, for any reason based on discrimina-*
*tion of any kind, when such pain or suffering is inflicted by*
*or at the instigation of or with the consent or acquiescence*
*of a public official or other person acting in an official*
*capacity. It does not include pain or suffering arising only*
*from—inherent in or incidental to—lawful sanctions.*

There are many similarities between torture and other forms of
trauma, especially in the psychological, physical, and psychobiological sequelae of the events. However, important elements dis-
tinguish the torture experience from other types of trauma. In
discussing this distinction, I am referring to torture in general,
not just political torture. In contrast to traumatic events in general, the torture experience is characterized by absolute control,
purposeful breakdown of the will, unpredictability, and isolation.

The first important difference between torture and other
types of traumatic events is the complete control of the perpetrator over the victim, who feels absolutely impotent and helpless. It is now widely understood that the purpose of political
torture is not to extract information or to obtain a confession.
The effort to get information is simply another way to demonstrate to the victim how helpless he or she is (Johnson, 1996).

Second, observations such as the fact that torture frequently
continues long after all information has been given, or long after
information has lost its value, and the opinion of military au-
thorities that torture is a poor source of information, suggest
that torture is not perpetrated to obtain information or a confession. The treatment and study of survivors of political torture
during the past twenty years has yielded some important information about its purpose (Vesti and Kastrup, 1995). Professionals working with torture survivors agree that torture is an

intentional and systematic attempt to break the victim's will, to destroy his or her humanity and identity. Thus political torture often serves to eliminate outspoken community leaders, making them appear weak and subdued. It also creates a climate of fear that produces a sense of apathy and undermines political opposition. This breaking down of the victim further distinguishes torture from other violent and traumatic experiences.

A third differentiating factor is the unpredictability of the victim's situation. Domestic violence, combat, and some forms of child abuse and sexual abuse have a certain degree of predictability. Unpredictability of one's situation, an integral part of the torture experience, is exploited by the perpetrator. A fourth factor differentiating torture and other traumatic events is the isolation of the victim, who generally lives through the ordeal alone.

## POLITICAL TORTURE AND OTHER FORMS OF TORTURE

Political torture is not the only form of torture. The experiences of adult survivors of childhood torture and of children who have been tortured are also contained within the above definition of torture. A child subjected to unpredictable, sadistic, and ritualistic forms of abuse is also helpless and dependent on the perpetrator. A survivor of this type of abuse has also lived through a systematic breaking down of his or her spirit and sense of self. The abuse is unpredictable and the victim is alone, without any social support. Yet although childhood torture and political torture have certain aspects in common, there are important theoretical and observational differences.

A young child attempts to develop a sense of self at the same time that his or her sense of self is being assaulted. This is very different from the experience of a survivor of political torture, who generally is older and has a more developed sense of self.

The perpetrators of political torture are, generally, strangers. Even though brainwashing techniques are frequently used, the survivor, for the most part, knows who the enemy is. In sharp contrast, the perpetrators of a child's abuse are also the child's caretakers, who masquerade in the community and to the child as providing the love and caring the parental role implies.

A survivor of political torture usually has led a relatively normal life, which is then disrupted by an extreme event that threatens his or her very existence. In contrast, a survivor of childhood torture knows of no way of life other than to live with terror and to find adaptive survival strategies.

Survivors of both forms of extreme abuse generally suffer in isolation. However, a survivor of political torture probably has had experiences of social support. A survivor of childhood torture is unlikely to know that such a thing as social support exists. Social support is something new that they slowly learn about in the healing process.

In my work with adult survivors, I have observed some important and interesting differences. I am often amazed at how quickly survivors of political torture improve; how dramatically their symptoms abate in a short period of time. Based on my experience, I attribute this to the fact that the survivor had a sense of self prior to the traumatic event, a self that did not live in constant terror and fear of disintegration. A survivor of political torture generally also has many more resources to draw upon during the treatment process, such as positive memories from childhood. The attachment system, though shut down, because of the torture experience, usually has memory traces of positive attachment bonds, which can be reactivated in treatment. I think it is also important that a survivor of political torture finds it much easier to identify who the enemy is. Past positive experiences of human interaction provide crucial support during the healing process.

However, there are factors that contribute to the complexity of work with survivors of political torture as compared to survivors of childhood torture. One is the survivor's refugee status. Most of the survivors I have treated have not had legal status; they were in the process of obtaining asylum. This means that a person is in a constant state of disequilibrium, never knowing if he or she can count on the stability of putting down roots here or on the safety of not being sent back to the country where the torture occurred. In addition, survivors of political torture must navigate in an unfamiliar culture, transcend the language barrier, and find work that does not require them to have "papers." In my experience, this results in their feeling disorganized and overwhelmed. Their traumatic experience is compounded with adjustment to a foreign culture. Because of their uncertain legal status, they are often exploited by their employers. As a result, they often find it difficult to keep their therapy appointments.

Another difference between survivors of political torture and childhood torture, but not necessarily an impediment to treatment, is in their concept of psychotherapy. Survivors of childhood torture in my practice often come for treatment with some knowledge about what the process entails. Survivors of political torture come from many different cultures and generally do not understand this concept (the one exception being, perhaps, Argentina, where psychotherapy is at least as common as it is here). They come for relief of symptoms.

I also find that survivors of political torture, more than survivors of childhood torture, tend to fear that there is something dreadfully wrong with them; that they are going crazy. I believe this is because their continuous everyday experience of self has been disrupted by an extreme experience that forever changes how they perceive self and the world. Survivors of childhood torture, on the other hand, have constructed their world around survival of extreme experiences; to exist this way feels normal. Much of the healing process for survivors of childhood torture consists of discovering that this way of living is not normal.

Finally, survivors of childhood torture feel shame and guilt because of who they are. Their abuse becomes internalized. They interpret it as happening because they are inherently bad. Survivors of political torture are much more likely to experience guilt and shame for what they think they have done or not done (given names under torture, not protected family members or friends). Thus, in my experience, I have found that survivors of political torture are able to work through these feelings of guilt and shame more easily than survivors of childhood torture.

## EDITH'S STORY

Edith was referred to the Healing Center for Survivors of Political Torture,[2] where I was director of clinical services, in August of 1995. She began treatment with me and with a massage therapist/body worker. After she had been in treatment for one and a half years, a journalist asked if he could write about the Healing Center. In addition to interviewing some of the professionals, he asked to interview two of our clients; we were assured that all parties interviewed would have the right to approve the article (Miller, 1998). When asked, Edith was very eager to be interviewed. The interview was taped. In telling Edith's story I have drawn on her own words from the interview, just as she spoke them, in her own English. She struggled to speak in English as much as possible during the interview, although her psychotherapy was conducted in her native language, Spanish. Her English was sufficient for her to communicate with her body worker. It is important to note that, as we shall see, the telling of her story in this way could occur only after a good deal of therapy.

Edith is the oldest of nine children, born in El Salvador in 1967. Her family was poor and lived in the *campo*. She remembers almost nothing of the first five years of her life. "My bad life began when I was eight years old," she relates. Her country was at war with neighboring Honduras. "Everything started with the guns and fights, killing the children, ladies, old people. After that everything is afraid because I saw many people killed when soldiers kill them. Then somebody likes to kill me when I was fourteen years old. And that was terrible."

During the war with Honduras, Edith's family would flee to the mountains, sometimes for days. "My mom take me under the trees for sleeping. She put something over me because she not want the helicopters to see us because they kill everyone. Animals eat my body. Sometime we not eat for two or three days. After twelve years old, we never sleep in my house."

By the time Edith was fourteen El Salvador was embroiled in a brutal civil war. A well-known priest was assassinated on his way to her village for a religious festival. "Somebody run in the church to say, 'The Father is die!'" The soldiers killed him because he is a good man who helped all the children and poor people. Everybody come to that place where he's die, and after that the soldiers say everybody is a guerrilla, and that's why they have to kill everybody."

The area where Edith lived was, in fact, not part of the country controlled by the guerrillas. Her village was targeted by the military because of the liberation theology popular there, and because the priest who was murdered lived there and was well known for sympathizing with the needs of the poor.

Edith married at the young age of thirteen, naively believing that "the soldiers not rape you if you married." At fourteen she had just given birth to her first child when the soldiers entered her village.

"Thirty minutes after my girl was born, I get a shot in my stomach. They come in the house and they say, 'I going to kill you and then they kill all my neighbors around my house.' Her mother escaped with Edith's newborn child. For two days Edith lay wounded with no food, water, or medical attention.

The soldiers returned. "They say, 'Oh, you not die? Why you not die?' Then they take me and make me walk. I had all my insides torn up. It hurt three times more than to have a baby."

For a week, Edith was held captive by the military. She was given no food, water, or medical attention. The soldiers sadistically forced her to look at numerous people they had murdered and repeatedly threatened to kill her.

Edith still wonders "why they didn't finish it." Instead, the soldiers threw her out on a road, where a *campesino* (farmer) found her. She was transported to a hospital in San Salvador, where surgery was performed on her stomach. She was dangerously weak, and at this time, Edith believes she was given a choice whether or not to go on living.

"I remember when I die. You must believe me. One night— like somebody hold my feet. Something is out of my body. I see the body; it is mine. I go up, up, and it is dark, and I see angels pointing this way and that way, and I go in the middle. It is beautiful. But I not see my girl. My mom take the baby and then I get a shot. When I went up, I cry there and I say, 'I like to see my girl grow up and now I say I live for my children.' I cry there and boom! I am back in my body. It was bad when I come inside my body."

Edith thought that everyone would appreciate her because of the ordeal she had survived. Instead, after a brief period of tender, loving care by a cousin, her ordeal continued. A cousin who lived in San Salvador took her to his home and cared for her "like a baby." She was so weak she could not see, nor walk without holding on to things. This cousin holds a special place in her heart; she weeps whenever she speaks of him.

Two weeks later, her husband's family came and forcefully took her to their house, to be reunited with her husband and baby. She could barely take care of herself, yet they made her clean and wash clothes. Edith claims that she and her children were mistreated by her husband's family off and on for years while living in El Salvador.

In 1988, seven years after her harrowing brush with death, Edith escaped from her war-torn country to find refuge in the U.S. She left her two children with her mother in El Salvador. Her journey overland with *un señor* (a "coyote," a man paid to bring refugees to the U.S.) was difficult and frightening. As she and her husband worked to earn the money to bring her two children here, she constantly worried that they would be killed by death squads in El Salvador. The children traveled eleven days by sea to join their parents in the U.S.

Only after Edith's arrival in the U.S. was the bullet removed from her abdomen. She and her husband filed papers seeking asylum in 1989. When Edith entered treatment with me in 1995, she and her family were still living in limbo.

## THE TREATMENT PROCESS

When Edith began treatment with me in August of 1995, she was twenty-eight years old. She had been in the U.S. for seven years; it had been fourteen years since her persecution by the *Fuerzas Armadas* of El Salvador.

Edith has long dark hair, dark eyes, and is of medium height and weight. She is articulate and expressive. She speaks to me in fast-paced Spanish, occasionally throwing in a word or two of English. She impresses me as being very intelligent. She makes good eye contact and is highly interactive with me; the only exception is when she comes to her sessions in a disorganized, withdrawn state of shock.

Both her developmental history and traumatic past are revealed in her body structure. Characterologically, her body has a high energetic charge, which is constricted at the surface and compressed by muscular contractions at the waist, neck, and shoulders. Thus, the trunk of her body tends to be overcharged (too much energy), while her head, pelvis, arms, legs, and feet tend to be undercharged with energy. Much anger is held in her body, which belies her soft appearance. Her impulses are constantly held in check or choked off. She has a feeling of being trapped; she suppresses her anger and self-assertion. She generally feels burdened and under pressure; she endures stress by pleasing others and compromising her own needs. Her capacity to persevere and push through adversity are characteristics that, in my opinion, helped her survive her ordeal.

The oldest of nine children, Edith has always had a close relationship with her mother, and describes herself as a very obedient child who always did what her mother expected of her. The characteristics described above are reflected in the way that she endured her tortuous ordeal and subsequent reenactments. This is also how she currently lives her life—always feeling under pressure, bearing the burden of the responsibilities of her marriage and her four children, overworking to support her children, and feeling intensely loyal to her husband, children, and employers.

Also structured in her body are the results of her shock trauma experiences. When she entered treatment, Edith's diaphragm was contracted, seriously restricting her breathing. Energy was frequently drawn to the center of her body and up into her head, resulting in a shock state in which she became immobilized to the point of hardly being able to move at all, even though her nervous system remained highly activated. She experienced a great deal of tension in her abdomen and neck. The flow of energy to her pelvis and abdomen was impeded by contractions in the tissue. Her legs and feet were almost always cold.

In her own words, Edith's symptoms at this time were: "fear, wanting to escape, to flee. Sometimes I stay for three days in my room and I no want to see anybody and I don't want to live; I cry a lot and I see all that happen to me [referring to flashbacks]. My body like die; I can't move [referring to immobility]. I have problems in my stomach—I vomit after I eat." In addition, she struggled constantly with hyperarousal and feeling overwhelmed. Her menstrual cycle had been irregular for years; she had not had her period for seven months when she began treatment with me. Infrequent menstruation is something I have often observed in women survivors of political torture.

Before beginning treatment with me, Edith had been to a number of mental health professionals. She described how, in her most recent therapy, she flooded with emotion, feeling increasingly out of control: "I don't want to come; when I tell her everything, I get sick; I cry and stay in my bed and I no want to do anything. When I have appointment again, I no want to go."

During my first meeting with Edith, I was struck by how frightened, desperate, tentative, and ambivalent she appeared to feel, as though she were ready to bolt out the door at any moment. At the same time, I was drawn to her apparent innocence, sweetness, and authentic charm.

In her first session I carefully educated Edith about trauma, making sure that she understood that she had lived through some extraordinary events, and that the problems she described were common for people who have suffered such extreme experiences. Describing to me how she struggles daily with her symptoms, feeling overwhelmed, suffering flashbacks, and vomiting, she expressed hopelessness that anyone could help her. I responded that it sounded as though she feels as if a monster lives inside her that at times gets out of control. She smiled and nodded, apparently relating to this idea.

I told her that she did not have to talk about what had happened to her right now—she could do that in her own time (I had reports from her lawyer and former therapist, so I knew her history). What we were going to do first was to help her feel better, to help her feel more in charge of her body. Had I not known how to work on a body level, I do not know what I would have done with Edith. Although desperate for help, at the same time she did not want to talk about her past or current life.

While she was sitting, I asked her to notice how she was breathing. She realized how shallow her breath was. I suggested that she put a little pressure on her feet, so as to feel the support of the floor when she inhaled, and then let all the air out when she exhaled. This simple intervention had a calming effect and facilitated the movement of energy downward into her pelvis, legs, and feet, resulting in her feeling connected with herself and with the ground. We then did the same thing as Edith stood with her feet shoulder-width apart, knees bent. When the tension in her body seemed to interfere with the movement of energy, I asked her to exaggerate the tensions. I asked her to notice what she was aware of as she did so, and to slowly come out of the exaggeration. As we worked she would at times say, "*Funciona*" (it works). It was evident that she was feeling much less anxious, more trusting, and more confident in herself.

She began to talk to me about what had happened to her. She would tell me a little bit and then stop, and we would work some more physically. Then, on her own, she would tell me a little bit more and then stop. She was clearly pacing herself as we kept all that was happening grounded in her body. By the end of the first session, she had related parts of her story, without feeling the least bit anxious or out of control.

Initially her treatment plan included weekly sessions with me and a massage therapist/body worker (hands-on work). After four months of treatment it became evident that there were serious problems in Edith's marriage and with her two oldest girls (who were also highly traumatized, having been born in El Salvador). Therefore marital therapy for Edith and her husband by another treatment provider was included in the treatment plan. About nine months later her two oldest girls were included in the treatment process by a third psychotherapist. I included the two oldest daughters in sessions with Edith five times. Attempts were made to involve Edith's husband—also highly traumatized from the war—in individual treatment, without success. Because of additional stress in her life, which made it difficult for Edith to maintain the stability she had achieved in therapy, ten months into her treatment she was referred to the center's psychiatrist for a medical evaluation and was put on a low dose of medication.

During the initial phase of treatment the focus was on building trust, helping Edith sense that she had some control over what happened in her body, and facilitating her awareness of her sensations and feelings. In this way, she learned to recognize when she was beginning to feel overwhelmed or immobilized. I continued to educate her about how the problems she lived with in her current life related to her traumatic past, in order to counter her belief that there was something terribly wrong with her—that she was crazy.

Over the course of the first ten sessions, Edith reported—and I observed—a steady improvement in her symptoms. During this period she vacillated between feeling some stability, more hopeful, and more in charge of her body, and feeling very disrupted and overwhelmed.

## SESSION 4

After a month of treatment, although still feeling ambivalent about coming to therapy, Edith reported that she had been feeling much better. She said that she had been working with her breathing and with grounding at home between sessions and noticed that it helped her to feel less overwhelmed and anxious. Mostly she worked lying down, doing what we did in the sessions—intensifying how she is holding on to her breath and then releasing, exhaling into her lower abdomen, bouncing her pelvis, and then kicking to move the energy down into her legs and feet.

She told me that at times she felt very scattered and disorganized (overwhelmed) when she thought of all the things she had to do. Then she would notice that her body contracted, her breathing became shallow, and she would feel so totally drained of energy that she could do nothing to bring herself out of this state. This reflected a great deal of learning on her part. She was becoming aware of how she induced a state of immobility (freezing) by how she talked to herself and by what she did physically.

She was also noticing how particular external events precipitated this state of freezing. For instance, she related an interaction with her two oldest girls and her husband, which left her feeling helpless about how to solve the girls' problems. The incident triggered a state of feeling overwhelmed by her despair, rage, helplessness, and fear. She found herself in what (with my help) she now identifies as *el pozo* ("the well," referred to in the literature as "the black hole of trauma"). She felt weak, unable to move—she called this "feeling lazy." She called me as soon as she was able to get up from her bed, but did not leave a message. Still, to reach out to someone from this state was a big step for her. Soon thereafter, she was able to take the next step and leave a message when I did not answer the phone.

We worked physically with this state of immobility that Edith called "feeling lazy" in order to increase her awareness of how she goes into it and how she can come out of it. I also explained to Edith that as she works with this organization on a physical level, the tissue in her body is learning that there is another way to be; this seemed to make sense to her. I asked her to imagine that she was back in the incident with her daughters and husband, so that she could feel herself start to go into the shock state. As she sensed herself on the edge of going into this state, I suggested that she—voluntarily and with conscious control—go more deeply into the freezing and notice what was happening as she did. Then, I asked her to slowly come back out by releasing the contractions.

She felt how she cut off her breathing by constricting her diaphragm, how she squeezed her head and eyes, tensed her neck and shoulders, and how in doing this she began to dissociate from me, from the present. She reported not feeling much in her legs and feet. As she released the contraction, she came back into contact with me, her breathing deepened, and she could feel more in her legs and feet. We repeated this release process a number of times. Each time she became more aware of her sensations, and also of other events which have thrown her into this shock state.

To ensure that she left the session grounded in the present and feeling her own support, Edith did the following with my instruction: She stood with her knees bent, leaning slightly backward into an arch (as this stress position is called in bioenergetics). Then, standing erect, she slowly shifted her weight from one foot to the other. She then bent down into a squatting position and slowly straightened her legs, pushing her feet hard against the floor. I encouraged her, as usual, to use these interventions at home when it felt right for her.

During this session I was struck with the extent of the changes in her body. It was much easier for Edith to open her breathing, compared to my first session with her. Her abdomen was much more open; her vomiting had decreased markedly. It took very little time and effort for the energy to move down into her legs and feet; they were beginning to feel warm rather than cold all the time.

## SESSION 8

Edith arrived at her session feeling very disrupted and overwhelmed. It was clear to me immediately that she was in a state of shock.

She came into the room, lay down on the couch, turned her face away from me, and covered her eyes. I asked her to tell me what she was experiencing. She said that she felt empty, lazy, didn't even want to breathe, and felt cold. Fortunately, we had established a base of experience in working with this state of immobility when she was not actually in shock, so that she was maintaining some awareness and some connection with me. I asked her to intensify everything that she was doing and then to release the exaggeration. After doing this about four times, Edith took a deep breath, looked at me, and said, "I am back." She then entered a state of sadness, punctuated by flares of anger.

She told me that yesterday one of her youngest daughters had been slapped by a neighbor woman who was having an argument with her husband outside in the street. Apparently the two children looked at them while walking by, and the woman ran over and slapped one of the girls. Edith called the police, who did nothing. This was a potent trigger for her: Someone she loved was harmed (reminding her of all the violence in her country), but no one did anything to help (also reminiscent of the violence in her country). As we processed this, she began to feel less helpless. She decided that she would insist that her husband go with her to talk to the woman, and that she would also file a police report. She did follow through with this and felt empowered by doing so.

While processing this, Edith expressed how confused she often feels by the rapid shifting of feeling she experiences. She feels like two persons—one who is normal and one who, when something happens (like the incident reported above), feels like there is something terribly wrong with her. I explained to her again that this happens when a person has experienced something so extreme and traumatic as she did; that things that happen in the present can trigger her into what is called a trauma reaction, meaning that she goes into a state in which she is in the past, reliving what happened to her. She was slowly beginning to integrate this knowledge. However, as with other trauma survivors, I found that I needed to repeat this information over and over again.

Edith then told me that she was also very upset because she found out that she could not go to El Salvador to visit her mother, who was ill. Since she did not yet have asylum, she would not be able to reenter the U.S. if she left. As she talked about this, she began to contract again. We worked with her breathing and releasing the contraction, and she entered a more relaxed state in which she simply felt her sadness and anger.

Then Edith did an interesting thing, to be repeated in following sessions. She suddenly jumped up off the couch and began to put on her shoes, saying that she had to go. I looked at my watch and pointed out that we had half an hour of the session left. She seemed thrown by this and at first persisted in wanting to leave. As I slowed her down and asked her to pay attention to what was happening, it became clear to both of us that she was experiencing an impulse to flee—an impulse that was locked into her nervous system due to the many impulses to flee that could not be completed during her captivity. She had been held in the mountains, out in the open, not in a cell. There had been many moments when she wanted to run, but knew that she would be killed if she did. She then told me that she often flees when something happens at home that upsets her. She just runs out of the house, with no destination in mind. Or she will run out of the house, get into the car, and drive around for hours. Over the course of a number of sessions, we worked through this fleeing impulse by carefully tracking her bodily experience and allowing her nervous system and reflexive responses to slowly unwind.

Her work during this session led to an important insight that Edith came to on her own. She said that she felt like a prisoner inside herself; that she felt trapped. She talked of not having freedom during her whole childhood, because of the violence surrounding her. Then she had been taken prisoner. Even now she did not have the freedom to visit her mother. She was able to realize how the sense of feeling trapped like a prisoner still lived inside her, even though it was no longer a reality in her life. She understood that she brought a traumatic sense of being trapped into current situations: She felt trapped in her marriage, trapped by all the demands of her busy life, at times even trapped by her psychotherapy.

At the end of the session, Edith lingered in my office, looking at pictures and various things, asking me about them, as though she did not want to leave. This brought home even more clearly to her and to me how the fleeing response had no relation to her current reality (i.e., she did not really have to be anywhere else and did not really want to leave my office).

About five months into her treatment process, Edith began to report important shifts in how she was experiencing herself. By January of 1997, she was much more stable and organized in her life, she felt more in charge of what happened in her body, and she had integrated a healthier frame around her traumatic experiences.

During this time, Edith frequently missed sessions or canceled at the last minute. At one point, when working with her fleeing impulse, she insisted on coming to sessions only once every two weeks. Her reason was that she had too many other things to do. Indeed, her life is very demanding; in addition to working full-time, she takes most of the responsibility for maintaining the home and caring for the four girls. However, it was clear to me that her need to control her treatment process, to feel free to come and go, was a crucial part of her transference, which I needed to work with carefully. For Edith, at this juncture, I was the potential captor, and it was essential that I agree to her treatment plan.

Edith's trauma-specific transference occurring throughout the treatment cast me in many roles: the enemy who could entrap her; the perpetrator who she feared would make her relive her painful memories; the failed protector who did not respond when she reached out and called me but did not leave a message; and the longed-for rescuer who could solve all her problems. Understanding her transference reactions let me avoid acting on my countertransferential feelings. However, I certainly experienced a wide spectrum of feeling responses: rage at the inhuman treatment Edith had endured; frustration when she needed to hold me at arm's length while at the same time feeling desperately in need of help; helpless when unable to find solutions to her domestic problems; feeling overly protective of her, alternating with wanting to emotionally distance myself when she related the gruesome details of her torture.

By the fifth month of treatment Edith had established a strong, trusting bond with me. She was able to come more consistently to her sessions. She would call me when she found herself in a trauma reaction between sessions and leave me a message. She saw me more realistically as someone who would do all that I could to help her with the current problems in her life, but that there were limits to what I could do.

## SUMMARY OF SESSIONS 12, 13, 14

After five and a half months of treatment Edith consistently reported feeling much better, although she felt bewildered by her recovery. She said that she was not vomiting, her body was not contracting and freezing, her feet felt warmer, and she was able to stop herself from becoming lost in a flash-back when something triggered her. In one session she related that she had had a car accident and had handled it "like a normal person," meaning that she did not go into flashbacks, as had been her previous experience with disturbing events such as this.

She was experiencing her rage differently. Initially her rage was dissociated and would erupt inappropriately with her husband and daughters, or she would collapse, cry, and withdraw when she felt angry. Now, she explained that she would cry a little when angry, but then she was then able to feel the rage and stay in contact with the feeling. When it passed, she would feel very good. As is common with most trauma survivors, Edith had been reluctant to talk with anyone about the horror she had experienced. Now she was sharing her traumatic past with others. This included talking with her husband and daughters and educating them about trauma in the way that I had educated her.

Edith became even more motivated in her treatment. She knew that it was helping her and began to feel very hopeful that her future included more than just struggle and suffering. Edith said that many people were telling her that she looked much better, and indeed she did. Her eyes were bright and full of energy, her skin had more color, her hair (which had been falling out at the beginning of treatment) looked healthier and had stopped falling out, and she was having regular menstrual periods. In general, she looked and felt more alive. Edith was becoming more aware of her strength, something I had stressed from the beginning of treatment. She could integrate the knowledge that she had to have been very strong to survive what she did and to manage her life as she does now.

Edith initiated the next phase of treatment by beginning to share in more depth the details of her torture experience. At times she would express fear about remembering what had happened to her. I assured her over and over again that she could remember just a little at a time, and that it was possible to do this without flooding. At Edith's request, I had contacted her lawyer about her anxiety over her asylum application, submitted eight years earlier. This stage of therapy coincided with her lawyer initiating the asylum process. Needless to say, facing an interrogation interview by Immigration brought much of her traumatic past to the surface.

## SESSION 15

At the beginning of the session Edith stated that she was still feeling much better, even though she was experiencing a great deal of fear about the coming asylum interview. When she thought about her imprisonment, she began to reexperience how she had been interrogated by the soldiers during her captivity. She told me how painful it is to talk about what had happened and not be believed; she anticipated that the agent would doubt her story. As Edith talked, her body contracted and she began to go into immobility; she teared up, but stopped the tears. She was sitting on the couch. I sat next to her and placed my hand on her back, after asking her permission to do this. I asked her to bring her attention to what she was doing physically: "What are you noticing in your body right now?"

"Squeezing in my chest and my eyes," she replied.

"So, as you put your attention on the squeezing, what else do you notice?"

"There is a knot in my stomach."

We continued this way until her breathing began to open up, and she began a soft rocking motion with her body. She reported feeling "something in her legs," and we both observed micro-movements in her legs. She then looked me in the eyes and began talking again. She was now calm and present. As she continued, at times I would slow her down by referring her back to her bodily experience.

She talked about her anguish when she was forced to view many, many bodies of people who had been massacred by the soldiers. She told me that she had been taken before death squad members and told that if any one of them said that he recognized her, she would be killed. She wondered how people could be so cruel to others. While realizing that this experience had changed her life forever, she also reminded herself that she felt more hopeful about her life. Here she was weaving between the trauma vortex and the healing vortex. She would touch the edge of the freezing response while reporting some of the grisly details, and then move into a parasympathetic mode while talking about how strong she now knew she was, about her hope for the future, and about her belief that she survived for a reason. At the end of the session, while grounding on her feet to assure herself that she left feeling fully present, she mused about how she knew herself as two persons—one who feels good and feels that life is good, and the other who goes into "the well," feels terrified, and wants to die. She suggested to herself that she would not have to be this second person during her immigration interview.

The interview did, in fact, go very well. Edith said later that it seemed strange, because the interviewer was a woman and was very nice to her. She did have to recount the details of the violence she experienced and felt like crying, but held it back. Later she experienced some fallout. It sounded as though she was close to going into shock and into flashbacks, but she managed to bring herself out of this and back into the present. I found her self-management remarkable, given the degree to which this experience was triggering for her. It would be almost four months before she would learn that the whole family had been granted asylum.

The latest phase of treatment has been challenging to both Edith and me. The problems in her family intensified to the point that for a period of time Edith lived at the home of her employer, who had generously provided her with her own room. She would go home after school to spend time with her girls and then return to spend the night at the her employer's. For a time I did a great deal of social work—exploring all possibilities of getting help for her two oldest girls, who were skipping school and had become involved with gangs.

160

In her treatment we have emphasized helping Edith learn more about how to take care of herself in the midst of her stormy home environment. We processed the problems she was dealing with at home and worked physically to help her maintain her stability and to stay grounded with all that was happening. A related theme has been to help her see how, being unable to mobilize her assertiveness, she falls into the victim role, even with her husband and daughters.

Here is an example of how we worked somatically to help her step out of the victim role. Edith came to her session feeling disorganized, upset, and helpless. She sat in a chair in a collapsed posture. When I asked her to notice what was happening in her body, she reported that she felt fear—butterflies in her chest and knots in her stomach. As she focused on these sensations, and we slowly tracked how the sensations changed, her fear subsided. She took a deep breath and sighed. As she began to tell me what had happened, the fear sensations returned. I stopped her and asked her to attend to these sensations again. We did this a number of times, until she felt more energy in her body, pulled herself up out of her collapsed posture, and told me how angry she was with her two oldest girls. In addition to acting out by skipping school, they had played some cruel jokes on their mother.

Edith readily falls into the victim role with her daughters, who are increasingly exploitive. She felt appropriate anger as she related all that had transpired. She began to problem-solve in an assertive way, thinking of various solutions to the problems presented by the girls. Most importantly, she was feeling her own power and she could see how different the picture looked when she had energy to back her up.

The family problems continue. Edith gets knocked off balance at times, but does quite well regaining her stability. She knows that she is doing all that she can to resolve the problems; the rest is up to the other family members.

She acknowledges how far she has come in the interview with the journalist: "I don't feel fear very often now; not like before, like somebody going to kill me. I don't see all that happen to me in my head. Now when I talk about what happened to me I get better. But sometimes when I can't solve problems I want to die." Musing about how people often die from much less serious things, she added, "I have a baby, get shot, not eat for many days—it's amazing. That's why I think my body is strong. I love my body; I love myself. Now I am better and sometimes life is beautiful and sometimes I fight to live."

Speaking of the bond she has established with me, "When I have big problems I have Maryanna in my mind, because she believe and she understands what my feel is and I know she love me. I come here and I tell her everything." Touching the spiritual realm, she says convincingly, "God left me here for a reason; he gave me the life back to tell my story to those who don't believe."

# Chapter Eight

———— ❧ ————

## HANAH'S STORY:
## A SURVIVOR OF CHILDHOOD TORTURE

"What was I like when I came to you nine years ago, and how do you see me now?" asked Hanah. I answered truthfully, as I always do. She seemed satisfied with my answer. I then suggested that she answer her own question. In her characteristic manner she leaned back and closed her eyes, resettled her doll, Sweetie, on her lap, smiled, and said, "When I came to you I felt like a scared little grey mouse. I now feel like a strong opinionated crone. I feel so grateful to my 'kids' who did so much of the work."

Hanah's diagnosis was dissociated identity disorder, previously called multiple personality disorder. Hanah then told me what she was seeing in the images of her "inside kids." She saw a meadow where she, an adult, sat with me on a bench. The "core baby" is sometimes in her lap and sometimes in mine. The Spokesperson is sitting between us. No other "inside people" are visible. "Am I going to integrate?" she asked, her eyes wide with fascination.

"Yes, Hanah," I replied, "perhaps you are going to do that unmentionable thing—integrate." Hanah had maintained that she would never integrate. At one time years ago, she did not even want to hear the word spoken. Hanah did indeed completely integrate in the next few months.

Three months after the date of this session, at seventy-six years of age, Hanah died of cancer. I am still grieving her death as I write her story. I wonder if I will be able to do justice to this incredible person. I think of her as a truly great spirit; I miss her. We made an excellent team. Our relationship was exquisite and very complex; one that is difficult to put into words. I was certainly her mother—the good mother of all her "inside people." But, in an interesting and unusual way, she was also my mother. She was an older, wise woman, who loved and appreciated me and expressed her fond feelings for me openly, rather like the good mother I never had. Her heart was still open, even though she had lived through as serious an abuse history as I have ever heard. It seemed that everyone who met Hanah loved her.

## HANAH'S LIFE

Hanah was born in Vienna, Austria, to an upper-class Jewish family. She had one sister two years younger than she and two stepsisters, fifteen and seventeen years older. Her family presented to the world an image of respectability, culture, and money. They had gardeners, chauffeurs, butlers, nannies, and cooks. "My mother was considered to be one of the most beautiful women in Vienna and everyone seemed to like her," Hanah stated over and over again in her therapy. She was always attempting to reconcile this image of her mother with the experience of her mother she carried inside her. During her therapy she began to refer to her mother as "the crazy lady," never as "Mother" or as her mother.

After working with Hanah for a number of years, my impression was that her mother also had multiple personality disorder or dissociated identity disorder. Her mother's brutality toward Hanah and the image she presented to the world were so consistent and so incongruent that, I believe, only someone with such extreme dissociation could have accomplished it.

Hanah was physically and sexually abused by both of her parents from a very young age, according to memories or memory fragments that emerged in treatment over the years. Hanah's memories always surfaced as implicit memory or as somatosensory experience, most often beginning with body sensations. The abuse by her mother was twisted and sadistic. Her father's sexual abuse of her was perverted and misguided, but did not seem to have the sadistic quality so characteristic of "the crazy lady."

As we wove the tapestry of Hanah's life from the fragments of memories that emerged over the years, a frightening picture began to take shape. It indicated that her mother's side of the family was part of a transgenerational cult, probably Satanic. She had memories of her mother, her grandmother, her grandfather, and her uncle (her mother's brother) in relation to the cult experiences, but never any of her father's involvement. Her uncle appeared to be the head of the cult and her primary abuser. My impression was that her mother abused her mostly outside of the cult.

I am quite aware that professionals who work in the area of abuse understand the possibility that memories clients produce in therapy may be symbolic of what happened, rather than what actually happened; i.e., that cult abuse memories may be symbolic of abuse of another nature. I remain open to this possibility. But, in Hanah's case, the memories arose in the process of treatment so implicitly, with such congruity among the various memories and memory fragments, and also seemed to be so similar to memories of cult abuse reported in the literature and by my other ritual abuse clients, that I have little doubt of the veracity of her story.

Hanah also manifested the classic self-doubt syndrome we have come to recognize as characteristic of clients who recover memories of past abuse. Hanah continuously doubted her own experience of remembering; she constantly would say, "This is not true; this can't have really happened. I don't want it to be true. How could this have happened?" It was clear that there were serious distortions in the details of what happened, as would be expected in the perceptions of a child in shock, or even an adult in shock, for that matter. In any case, one would have to conclude that something terrible had happened to Hanah during her childhood; that she had survived extreme abuse and had had almost no experience with a soothing, loving, nurturing adult.

It is ironic that Hanah's being Jewish probably saved her from even more extreme abuse later. Hanah's father anticipated the Nazi invasion of Austria and moved the family to Czechoslovakia. He had a factory in Czechoslovakia, and the family continued to live their upper middle-class lifestyle. However, the transgenerational cult was left behind in Austria. Hanah had no memories of cult experience after the age of about twelve to thirteen. Her parents continued to be abusive, but the extreme torture she endured in the cult stopped.

Before Hitler's invasion of Czechoslovakia, Hanah's father sent his children to London, and soon followed with their mother and as much of his money as he was able to take. After finishing her schooling, Hanah worked in the Anna Freud nursery school. She married a German man and bore three children, two boys and a girl. When her children were small, her husband left her for another woman. She raised the children alone, with financial help from her former husband. When her children were grown, Hanah moved to the United States, where her mother, uncle, and sister already resided.

Hanah had no idea that she had "inside people" or that she harbored a horrible history of abuse until about 1988, four months after her mother died. She thought that she had had a happy childhood, except that she could remember nothing about it. She had been in psychoanalysis in London for two years, while in her teens, at her father's suggestion. She claims that in her analysis she literally said nothing, and neither did her analyst; she would lie down on the couch for fifty minutes and then leave. She remembers feeling too afraid to talk. Finally, after two years of therapy, her analyst told her that she could do nothing more for her, and that they should terminate the therapy.

In 1984 Hanah began treatment for eating disorders in an inpatient clinic. She was a binge eater and quite overweight. During her hospitalization, she produced a great deal of art work, and symbols of her abuse began to spill out over the pages of drawings and paintings. At the time she had no idea what they meant. However, she became motivated to enter treatment with a psychotherapist in 1985. About three years into her treatment, and after her mother's death, memories of abuse began to arise. Shortly after this she began to realize that she had "inside people" with distinct personalities, behaviors, names, and histories.

The relationship with her therapist was Hanah's first experience in forming a loving, trusting relationship with another human being. She opened up emotionally and allowed herself to become deeply involved in this relationship. In 1989, Hanah's psychotherapist announced that she was getting married and moving to Canada, realizing Hanah's worst fear. Hanah felt devastated and suicidal. She continued therapy for the eleven months before her therapist left, and then saw her every few months, when her therapist made return visits, for the next year. Hanah felt unable to let go of her therapist. It seemed impossible to her that she could bond with a new therapist.

## THE TREATMENT PROCESS

### PHASE ONE: BUILDING TRUST AND RESOURCES

Two months before her therapist was to depart, Hanah was referred to me by a friend of hers. I can still clearly see the short, overweight, grey-haired woman, with such an interesting and unusual face, eyeing me suspiciously, while at the same time engaging me with her authentic charm. I liked her instantly and was captivated by the aura of mystery that seemed to surround her. She was an extremely smart and very clever woman, although she didn't think of herself as such.

Hanah and I met three times a week. For the first two years of treatment with me, Hanah focused on her grief over the loss of her previous therapist and her difficulty learning to trust me. I attempted very little work on a body level during this time, as it was far too threatening to her. If I asked a question, such as, "What are you aware of in your body right now?" she would adamantly and stubbornly reply that she did not even want to hear the word "body."

"I hate my body," she would say frequently. "It is dirty and disgusting."

Slowly Hanah began to bond to me, as she let go of her former therapist. She would express worry and concern when I went out of town. She was able to reach out and to call me between sessions when she was struggling in the trauma vortex. Her "inside people" began to communicate directly with me instead of through Hanah. More and more of them came out to meet me.

In working with people who have suffered undergone great suffering, the conventions of a middle-class therapy may be inadequate to contain the assault on the foundations of humanity itself. Such an assault calls on the deepest human response of the therapist, who may bypass therapeutic formalities. Thus, I found myself doing things with Hanah that I do not generally do with clients. For instance, I always answered questions the that Hanah asked me about myself, after exploring where the question was coming from. Her questions never felt intrusive or inappropriate, and we maintained strict boundaries around the therapy at all times.

She is the only client with whom I have shared my own trauma history. This occurred only after Hanah had asked, we had processed this for a time, and when Hanah felt sure that she was ready to hear my story.

Later in treatment Hanah told me how important responding truthfully to her questions had been in her healing process. I did not think about this rationally at the time, but did it because it felt right. Now, as I look back, I think that Hanah grew up with such a sense of confusion about what was real or not real that receiving truthful responses to her questions was very meaningful. It was significant in her learning to trust me and also to trust herself and her own reality.

I always gave Hanah phone numbers where I could be reached when I went out of town, even when I was teaching in such faraway places as Spain or El Salvador. It was as though her "inside kids" needed to feel that they had a link to me to help them tolerate my absence. We both knew that she probably would not call. I also held Hanah when she specifically asked me to. I sat next to her on the couch, put my arms around her, and held her tightly. Although I use touch with clients, I rarely find myself holding them. Later in her healing process Hanah stressed how important this had been for her. My holding her so that she could feel me was crucial in her becoming able to soothe herself at difficult times between sessions.

Hanah had developed a good observing ego even before she began treatment with me. She was able to observe her own transferential feelings for me. I always felt that I was learning from her how to treat her. However, the work was made less difficult for me because she could see that much of her feelings for me were related to her past. If I was a few minutes late to meet her in the waiting room, she was able to contain her feelings of rejection and dismissal without seriously believing that I experienced her as a burden.

Hanah's feelings for me probably covered everything I mentioned about transference and trauma in the above discussion. Her alters, who would come out and then recede, did believe their own feelings for me. But this was tempered by Hanah reemerging as the executive personality who ran the show. For instance, one of her alters believed at one time that I would be contaminated by her violent past, and that some harm would come to me because I was in close association with her. One of her alters, named Mary, believed that nothing bad or dramatic had ever happened in Hanah's life. She hated me for exploring Hanah's past with her.

My countertransference for Hanah grew over the years into feelings of love and respect for her. I found her challenging and always extremely interesting. Through the long years of processing so many devastating memories, I sometimes doubted my capacity to keep her from drowning in the trauma vortex. She was in so much pain at times that I was unable to avoid my own feelings of helplessness and hopelessness. I understood her feelings of not wanting to be here on this earth because of my own trauma history. She knew that I understood, and it was very meaningful for her.

We both knew that feeling that one does not want to be alive is not quite the same as feeling suicidal. However, at one point she was extremely suicidal, and she had the means to kill herself. She had been collecting sleeping pills prescribed by a doctor. I felt desperate. I was unable to even convince myself that someone in so much agony should want to live. I resorted to baring my heart to her, letting her know how much I cared for her, and how much I did not want her to die. It did result in her giving me the pills. This brought our relationship to a new level. Hanah's belief that no one could really care about her was penetrated, and she began to let in more of the genuine love that those who knew her felt for her. I was deeply affected by the experience. I reached a new level in my caring for her.

In the first two years of therapy with me, Hanah was relatively numb. She felt grief over the loss of her previous therapist
but she did not weep. In fact, Hanah could not cry tears. She
eventually learned to cry (make sobbing sounds), but no tears
flowed from her tear ducts. Her last wish, expressed shortly before her death, was that she would be able to cry tears before she
died. At times during her last months a few tears did leak down
her cheeks, but she never wept as one does ordinarily.

She felt anger about her abandonment by her therapist, but
it was constricted and generally turned inward. In fact, Hanah
was very disconnected from her body. In a detailed recording I
made in 1992 of her awareness of her experience, she reported
almost no body sensations; a few images, very little affect, some
behavior (mostly small movements, like hands twitching, a rocking motion); mostly meaning—thoughts and interpretations of
her experience. One of my intentions was gradually to shift her
awareness to include body sensations, affect, and behavior in an
attempt to help her reconnect with her bodily experience.

For those of us in the body-oriented psychotherapy world
Hanah's body structure would be considered as complex as she
was. There is nothing written about the body structure
of persons with dissociated identity disorder. However, one
would expect to see fragmentation in the body and other characteristics that result from neglect, deprivation, and abuse early
in life. Hanah's body structure had elements of the existence
structure or schizoid structure, the oral or need structure, and
the masochistic or will structure (Lowen, 1958; 1975; Keleman,
1985). The pupils of her eyes were always enlarged, and her eyes
were wide open as they would be in shock. She would frequently report that her hands felt as though they "did not go together" when she held them together. I could only surmise that her
hands felt as though they were touching someone else's hand
and not her own. Her head seemed too small for the rest of her
body. She was overweight with small hands and feet. A collapse

in the middle of her body was visible. Typical aspects of the shock structure were apparent. She was frozen in the diaphragm. She carried a great deal of tension at the base of her skull and in her neck. Her abdomen was in knots most of the time.

About five years into her treatment, when Hanah herself knew her "inside people," I suggested that she draw a map of them to see just who was there. She carried about thirty alters inside her. Some were integrated into other alters by the sixth and seventh years of treatment. The primary alters, who interacted with me and played a role in her healing, were the "three little ones," younger than eighteen months. Others were Fetti, who drove her binge-eating behavior; Anna, who criticized everything Hanah and I did together; Mary, who was in denial, and hated me for exploring Hanah's past with her; Tashi, who carried only positive memories; Rudy, who carried the rage; the Fantasy Girl, who emerged very late in treatment and held only good memories of the "crazy lady"; and the Spokesperson, who spoke for more and more of the others as the years passed. All of Hanah's alters had distinct personalities and well-defined appearances. When one emerged, I definitely felt as though I were talking with a five-year-old child or a thirteen-year-old girl.

Although I believe it important to mention Hanah's intricate and enigmatic inner world, I did not focus on her alters during her treatment. I focused on the issues with which she was struggling and worked with the issues through the alters. For instance, at one point it became clear that one child alter, Fetti, was very involved in Hanah's problem of overeating. Thus, it was necessary for me to get to know this alter, to get her to trust me and to come out and talk with me, in order to work effectively with Hanah's eating disorder.

Hanah referred to herself as "Hanah and the clan." She always used the word "we" instead of "I" or "us" instead of "me' when referring to herself, as is the case with most persons with dissociated identity disorder with whom I have worked.

Near the end of her treatment, awareness of a part of her that was never abused emerged, whom Hanah called "the core baby." Although she was not very aware of it while it was taking place, her many alters gradually integrated into one person, the Spokesperson, who spoke for all of the others. The one exception was the Fantasy Girl, who appeared during the last year of her therapy. She startled and upset Hanah tremendously, as she carried the few pleasant memories of the "crazy lady." I must admit that I became very attached to the Spokesperson, the last alter to integrate. There was something so sweet, so captivating, and so engaging about this alter that I missed her when she melted into just being part of Hanah.

During those first three years of treatment Hanah gradually gave up her fierce objection to her body and began to cooperate with me in using somatic interventions. One of the first things I was able to get her to do was to focus on her breath and to notice how far down the movement of energy went when she exhaled. At first the movement stopped in the area of her diaphragm; this was not surprising, given how frozen she was in this part of her body. However, over time the freezing began to melt, and the movement of energy on the exhalation went down to her abdomen, then her pelvis, and finally to her feet. This became a little game I played with her "inside kids," who delighted in seeing how far down the breath would go each time. She became open to feeling her feet on the floor and to putting some pressure on them when she inhaled. At times she would even stand and bend her knees in the typical bioenergetic grounding position and would become interested in watching the movement of energy descending to her feet.

I frequently asked Hanah what she was aware of in her body, attempting to increase her sensory awareness. At first she found this annoying but later she began to laugh about my persistent question and even felt gleeful when she could get the question in before I did. Her body awareness grew to where she was able to lean back, close her eyes, and track her sensations comfortably. She then learned to bring into consciousness her associations at other levels of awareness. For instance, while noticing tightness in her abdomen she might report feeling fear and then become aware of a memory or an image. Thus, after a few years of treatment Hanah was able to track her experience and keep it anchored in her sensate experience.

Another resource I used a great deal with Hanah was to ask her to slowly exaggerate how her body was organized and then to release the exaggeration, tracking her awareness as she did so. This intervention is an especially fine way of working with resistance and how it is organized in the body. It is also a way of making conscious what the client is doing unconsciously. As a person repeatedly exaggerates and releases what he is doing unconsciously, he gradually begins to feel more in charge of his body.

We worked with how Hanah somatically organized her fear and panic, helping her to slowly feel less victimized by these feelings. We also worked with how she organized to hold in her rage, so that she was more conscious of how she did this.

This approach was also helpful in working with her eating disorder. I would ask her to bring back a memory of the state she was in when she had binged. As she exaggerated and released how she was organized, she would get in touch with the feelings that she was stuffing down, i.e., anger and longing. Gradually, over years of treatment, Hanah was able to become more aware of her sensations of hunger and fullness and saw how eating did not fill up her longing or help her escape from her anger for long.

Hanah had almost no positive memories. In those first few years I would ask her to bring to mind a positive image or memory and sense the correlating feeling in her body. She did have one positive memory of dancing with her friend Annie at Annie's house, and how free and excited she felt. In relation to this memory she felt expansive in the tissue and tingling with the movement of energy through her body. A second image came to her of dancing in the moonlight. Embodying this image heightened the fluidity and expansiveness in her body. The positive memories, images, and corresponding sensory experiences served as sustaining resources when we were renegotiating the horrific memories that besieged Hanah.

Another enhancing resource was the rudimentary development of Hanah's spiritual life, which played an important function in her process toward the end of her life. She began by finding and frequently visiting a "sacred place" in nature—a particular tree and the surrounding area. I encouraged her in her endeavor to find peace in nature and inside her. She did very little that was tangible to evolve spiritually over the years, but in her quiet way she was growing markedly in the spiritual dimension. She later credited me for helping her to evolve this way, although I did little other than always talking frankly and openly with her about the metaphysical level of experience. Yet, by the end of her life she was well beyond me spiritually in the way she lived each day of her life.

Thus, by the third year of treatment Hanah had developed the following resources in her treatment with me: She had bonded with me and had other close relationships in her life. She was able to reach out to me and others in her life. Her "inside people" could communicate directly with me. She had made substantial progress in reconnecting with her bodily experience and being able to listen to her body, and she could use somatic interventions that I introduced. She had begun her evolution as a spiritual being. She was very intent on healing herself.

## PHASE TWO: THE TRAUMA VORTEX: BASIC ISSUES AND MEMORIES

The trauma vortex (Levine, 1991, 1997) includes all the undigested and unintegrated traumatic elements, such as traumatic memories, feelings of terror and rage, associated body sensations, and behavioral reenactments. The trauma vortex is dissociated from—that is, outside of—the normal stream of life experience. When swept into the trauma vortex, a person loses touch with other aspects of her experience. The person is flooded emotionally and retraumatized by reliving and reenacting the traumatic experiences. The healing vortex, a counter force, balances the force of the trauma vortex (Levine, 1991, 1997). Here exist the support and resources that aid the healing process. The healing vortex consists of healing memories and images, parasympathetic activity, positive thoughts, and innovative and expansive body movements.

In the second phase of treatment Hanah's basic issues became clarified. We worked on them, while at the same time we dealt with the memories that were to assail her for the next five years or so of treatment. Her fundamental problems included her disconnection from her body; her dissociation, resulting in many inside alters and the fragmenting of her experience; her lack of self-confidence and extremely low self-esteem. She had difficulty reaching out to others for support, and she could not let in the love and support offered by others. Her affect disregulation resulted in her being flooded and overwhelmed by her feelings. She could not experience pleasure or soothe and calm herself. In addition, she had a serious eating disorder.

During this phase of treatment we focused on many of these issues, such as reconnecting with her bodily experience. Maintaining her stability and not being swept off balance by the memories and events in her life was also an important area of focus, as was her capacity to relate to others and to take in their caring. Another aim of treatment was to help her learn to regulate and express her affect, especially her rage. She had to learn to trust herself. She was gradually learning to introject me and to be able to self-soothe. Slowly she achieved more clarity in her identity by becoming more integrated, i.e., far less dissociated and fragmented. We worked conscientiously on her eating disorder. This was the last thing to resolve, but toward the end of treatment, with no effort, she shed sixty pounds.

From nine extensive years of psychotherapy with Hanah, I would like to discuss how somatic interventions were helpful in working with two of her primary issues—her rage and her eating disorder. I will then demonstrate the importance of somatic work in integrating traumatic memories into a larger sense of self.

Because of the extreme abuse and humiliation Hanah had suffered her entire childhood, she harbored a murderous rage. Initially, whenever her rage would surface, she would constrict her body, especially her abdomen, shoulders, and neck, cover her mouth with both hands, and make a minute rocking motion. Her experience was self-hate, self-disgust, and fear. She wanted to hurt herself and sometimes scratched or cut herself between sessions. Her rage was overcoupled with fear (Levine, 1997); i.e. when rage surfaced, she instantly felt fear in association with the rage. This is not surprising because any protest against her childhood abuse had been brutally crushed.

One day Hanah came to her session reporting that the night before she had wanted to scratch her own skin off. She had, in fact, scratched herself, but only superficially. I asked her if she could bring back that state now with me. She closed her eyes and soon stated that she was feeling similar to how she had felt the night before. I asked her to focus on the scratching impulses. Her fingers made minute scratching movements. I instructed her to keep her awareness with the movement, while at the same time noticing anything else that came into her consciousness.

"We see my uncle," she said, "and the 'crazy lady.'"

"When you see the images of them, what else do you feel?" I

asked. She began to make small scratching motions in the air.

"We want to scratch their skin off; we want to tear them to pieces," she cried.

"Good, Hanah," I said. "You can fight back now. They hurt you terribly; you can fight back now."

Suddenly she collapsed, put both hands over her mouth, and said, "We're afraid."

"Where in your body do you feel the fear sensations?"

"Here in our chest and abdomen,"

"What else do you notice about them?"

"They are fluttery and jumpy," she said.

"Go back and forth between the fluttery fear sensations and the impulses to scratch in your hands," I instructed her. Moving between two components, such as two sensations, is one method of uncoupling overcoupled elements. As Hanah did this, the scratching sensations became dominant again. She felt her rage and the impulse to direct it outward.

We worked with the scratching impulses, the tendency to turn them inward, and the overcoupled fear response over many sessions. Gradually Hanah was able to experience her aggression as directed outward, rather than imploded, and to feel her rage and aggression without collapsing into fear.

Also working with her rage, we focused on a small rocking motion that Hanah often made when working through memories or when working with events happening in her life. At first, when I asked her to attend to this small movement, she would freeze and say that she couldn't do so, that it went away when I called her attention to it. Nevertheless, I persisted, and over time she was able to begin to join with this small movement whenever it emerged. Eventually, as she focused her attention on the small movement, the rocking motion grew larger; she would clench her fists and jaw and make a somewhat strangled sound. She was clearly angry. At times she would then freeze, and I would encourage her to be as aware as possible of how she froze and maintained the freezing. As she focused on how she froze, she would once again come out of the freezing and begin the rocking motion.

I surmised that in her tortured childhood Hanah often took to rocking when feeling full of rage, in an effort to soothe herself. Again, this took many sessions to fully work through. But finally Hanah was able to feel good, clean rage and anger and to sense her aggressive impulses uncontaminated by fear, freezing, constriction, and collapse. This working through manifested itself in her life so that she was able to take a stand for herself, set clear boundaries with people, and assert her own needs.

Somatic interventions also proved to be important in working with Hanah's eating disorder. Hanah was a binge eater. She would often begin eating at noon or in the afternoon and continue to eat until she went to bed. She was quite overweight, so that she could not exercise even by going for walks. Years earlier she had lost a good deal of weight when she entered an inpatient treatment program for eating disorders and then followed up by going regularly to Overeaters Anonymous. But when she began treatment with me, her eating was again out of control. It did not resolve until the last two years of treatment.

In her chaotic and brutal family, eating seemed to be the only area of her life where Hanah felt she had some control over her own body. She sometimes refused to eat. When she was old enough to get food on her own, she would sometimes stuff herself. Thus, the eating disorder was driven by an illusion of control. It was particularly associated with one alter named Fetti ("fat" in German). Fetti came out to meet me fairly early in treatment, but was hostile and suspicious of me for a long time. Gradually, Fetti became more motivated to know me and to find out how I might help.

This child alter was stubborn and confused about the eating problem. She felt frantic about being so out of control with the eating, while at the same time maintaining the illusion that it gave her a sense of control. She was very afraid that Hanah and I would deprive her of this overeating behavior, which was her domain of influence.

I worked with Fetti when she emerged or expressed a need to talk to me. I worked primarily in a cognitive-behavioral way to help her untangle the threads of her mixed-up thinking. Eventually she became friendly with both me and Hanah, and she merged into Hanah. Hanah was then more in charge of the eating behavior, because it was not being driven by a dissociated part of her.

I worked somatically with Hanah on her eating disorder. For instance, she would frequently come to a session and tell me that she had binged the last few days. I would ask her to close her eyes and bring back the state she was in when she began the binge eating "When we left your office we were thinking about food—about going to the supermarket and what we would buy."

"What are you aware of in your body, Hanah, as you remember this?"

"We feel empty."

"Where do you feel the emptiness?"

"Here," she says, putting her hand on her abdomen.

"Just notice the empty sensations, and we will see what comes next."

"The 'little ones' want to be with you all the time," she said referring to the three youngest "inside children." She was making a minute rocking motion, and I asked her to attend to it. The rocking motion became stronger. Hanah said, "We feel so angry that we can't be with you all the time; we were very angry when we went to the store."

"So you felt that deep longing and also anger."

"Yes, then we went home and I took out the bread. . . ." She went on to relate in some detail how she began the binge. I asked her what she was aware of in her body. She responded that she could not feel her body.

It became clear that she dissociated from her body when she ate, so that she could not feel the sensations of hunger or fullness. When I asked about her bodily awareness, even in the most basic somatic questions ("Can you feel your feet on the floor right now? Can you feel the weight of your hands in your lap?"), she became more aware of how her eating was an attempt to control—stuff down—her feelings of longing and anger. She also became more aware of how temporary this solution was and how bad she felt in her body after she had stuffed herself. This took many sessions over the course of several years, but gradually her awareness of all the details of this self-defeating behavior led to a resolution. It was neither sudden nor dramatic. She would just report that she had not binged for quite a while. She stated now and then that she was losing weight. Finally, it seemed clear that the binge eating had vanished for good, and Hanah had lost sixty pounds.

One particular memory fragment was very persistent in Hanah's experience over the years. It seemed that it was part of many, if not most, memories Hanah reconstituted. She referred to it as, "Those feelings between our legs." This was the sensation of hands sexually stimulating her to the point of being extremely uncomfortable. The feeling of being overstimulated sexually would just emerge at times for no apparent reason, both in sessions and between sessions at home. When it surfaced in sessions, I would work with it in the following way.

"We feel those feelings between our legs," Hanah said, squirming uncomfortably on the couch.

"What happens when you focus on them totally instead of trying to squirm away from them?" I asked. She put her attention totally on the sensations, and soon said, "They go away or become less."

"Good," I responded. "So just focus on the sensations and let's see what happens next." I saw micromovements in her hands and lower arms and called her attention to this. "Let that small

181

movement come through, Hanah." I also noticed micromovements in her legs and suggested she notice this also. Soon the micromovements in her arms and hands and legs expanded into a trembling, and I commented on the discharge of energy.

The movements become more pronounced. Hanah said, "We want to push them away; we want to kick." I encouraged her to let the pushing movement come through her arms and to allow the movement in her legs to grow into something that looked more like kicking. "We hate them," she said. "We want to push and kick them." As the movement settled down and the trembling through her limbs subsided, she reported that the "feelings between our legs are gone."

We worked through this scenario many times before the pushing and kicking impulses freely intervened when the feelings between her legs came. Eventually she no longer experienced these distressing sensations. However, this memory fragment was very persistent and troublesome. It took several years of attention to dissolve.

During Hanah's treatment we never made any attempt to retrieve memories from her past. Instead, her memories besieged her at times. She did not want to remember; she did not want to believe that what she remembered was true. Yet the memories came, always as implicit memory, most often beginning with body sensations and overwhelming affect. When it seemed that a memory was pressing to make itself known, I would schedule a two-hour session for Hanah to allow plenty of time to complete the process once we entered it. Soon Hanah's "inside kids" seemed to know when she needed a two-hour session. We both learned to trust them, since they were always right; something was indeed brewing inside.

I will attempt to relate how the memories made themselves known and how we renegotiated the material, keeping her experience anchored in her bodily experience, while allowing all levels of experience to be expressed. Keeping her connected to her bodily experience ensured that she not only stayed connected to herself, but to me and to the present as well.

One of her first and least horrific memories began with her experiencing the "feelings between our legs," along with a sense of feeling paralyzed and unable to move. I began working with her with these two bodily experiences. As she focused on the sensations of feeling paralyzed or the sensations of being sexually stimulated, she began to see images of herself at about age seven sitting on the steps of the veranda with the manservant, who had his arm around her and was fondling her. She experienced impulses of wanting to run and to push him away, but she immediately felt fear and became immobilized.

I asked her to focus on the fear sensations she said she felt in her chest, the constriction she sensed in her body, and the quietness of the immobility. As she did this she said she felt a "blank space." I replied that blanks are good—to just be with the blank space. She breathed more deeply and her body expanded some. I asked if there was an image that went with the expanded feeling. She said, "Yes, like we are growing wings and flying away."

I suggested that she keep focusing on her body. I could see her body expand and open up. She began to feel impulses to push and to run and little flares of anger. As I encouraged her to attend to these sensations, she said, "We want to push him away; we want to run away." As these impulses became stronger, she felt tremendous strength in her body and also justifiably angry about the violation. She made small pushing movements with her arms, and I could see micromovements in her legs.

"Just let the little movements come through, Hanah," I said. The pushing movement in her arms became a little stronger, and her legs began to tremble and shake, discharging much of the energy that had been held in her nervous system.

Images that emerged again and again in Hanah's memories, suggestive of the cult experience, were of a large dark basement room, a table with a marble top, people standing around in black hoods and gowns. Hanah recovered one cult memory in which one side of her labia minora was cut off, cut up, and offered to cult members to eat. She once was told by a gynecologist that she was missing one side of her labia minora. This is the only memory for which there is tangible confirmation, but it is a rather compelling confirmation.

One of Hanah's most horrible memories began with the bodily experience of congested lungs, rather like asthmatic symptoms. She was examined several times by doctors, but no cause could be found. The symptom persisted for about six weeks. She was becoming increasingly agitated during this time and was having difficulty maintaining her emotional stability. I finally decided that it might be part of a body memory and scheduled a two-hour session.

We began the work by simply focusing on the congested sensations in her chest. She became increasingly agitated, and I slowed her down by having her open her eyes, make contact with me and feel her feet on the floor. A shudder and trembling went through her body, indicating the discharge of a large amount of energy held in her nervous system. She took a deep breath, and I could see her body expand as her energy settled. She then began to cough and to complain about smoke and having difficulty breathing.

"There is too much smoke; we can't breathe; it's the pot; there's blood in the pot," she shrieked. Again I slowed her down and asked her to open her eyes and make contact with me and the present. She was shaking and trembling, and I suggested she just let the trembling happen and to notice the shaking. As she focused on her body, and discharged more energy, she calmed down rather quickly.

Soon she began to activate again. She had the image of being held up over the pot, which was boiling over a fire, and being forced to look in. She saw blood and body parts. I brought her back once again to the sensations in her body.

"We can't breathe very well; we are shaking all over."

She then froze and felt paralyzed. I asked her to just be with the paralyzed feeling in her body. She became quite immobilized, her eyes wide with fear. At one point she gasped and said, "They are going to cut off their heads; if we breathe, if we scream, they will cut off our head." She then reported images of two children being beheaded and their heads being kicked around like balls. She asked to hold my hands; she grasped them and sobbed, but without making a sound. I asked her to look at me and to tell me what she was experiencing in her body. "We have a knot in our throat," she replied.

"Focus on the knot, Hanah. See what happens as you do this."

"It starts to go away."

We did this a number of times—the knot returned, she focused on it, and watched it fade away. Finally, she broke into sobs, daring to make a sound. "I don't believe it," she wept. "It couldn't have happened. I should have been killed."

Hanah experienced a great deal of survivor guilt as a result of this memory and others. Her earlier experience in the cult included her terror that she, too, could be killed. However, at some point she realized that she was considered "special," having been born on Friday the thirteenth. It seemed that not only did the cult not want to kill her, but she was being groomed for a special place in it. Perhaps for this reason she was subjected to numerous events in which, even as a very small child, she was tricked into believing she had killed someone or had participated in the killing.

One such memory involved Aya, who was Hanah and her sister's nanny from the time that Hanah was born until she was seven years old. One day Aya disappeared, never to return again. Hanah simply remembers being told that she had gone away. A memory about what actually happened to Aya began with another body sensation that was relentless. It persisted on and off for weeks. It was a burning sensation around her neck, like a burning hot necklace. Hanah was mildly distressed about this; we were both very puzzled. We scheduled a two-hour session.

I began by working with the burning sensation, having Hanah focus on it. It became quite uncomfortable, so I brought her back into contact with me for a reprieve. We did some grounding, made some eye contact, and then she went back to the burning sensation. "He is putting it around my neck," she said finally.

"Who is, Hanah?"

"My uncle is; he is mad."

"Focus on the burning, Hanah, and tell me, why is he mad?"

"It is Aya," she cried out. "I killed Aya." As I slowed the process down, allowing the discharge of enormous amounts of energy to take place slowly, and making sure Hanah stayed connected to me in the present by keeping her anchored in her bodily experience, the following grisly picture emerged. However, it is important to note that the details were filled in slowly, over many more sessions.

Hanah is in a room with her uncle. He is fondling her, as was so typical, and then asks her if she wants to see Aya. Hanah feels full of excitement and expectation. He takes her into the next room. She sees Aya sitting on a table with her back to her; she has no clothes on. Her uncle hands Hanah a knife and tells her to plunge it into Aya's back. Hanah is horrified and cannot do it. Her uncle then takes the knife, puts it into Hanah's hand, places his hand over hers, and plunges the knife into Aya's back. As we processed the details over many sessions, it seemed clear that Aya made no noise and that there was no blood. My guess is that Aya was already dead, and this was an attempt to torture Hanah into thinking that she participated in the killing of her beloved nanny. It worked. She did believe it until after we had done months of reworking these images and body memories. Because she refused to do what he instructed her to do—plunge the knife into Aya's back—her uncle put a red-hot "necklace" around her neck that burned her, as punishment for disobeying him. This all happened in the presence of other cult members, according to the images that Hanah processed.

The burning sensation around her neck, associated with punishment, and her guilt for having harmed Aya were overcoupled, meaning that the burning sensation would surface, Hanah would feel like a terrible person, and would blame herself for Aya's death. It took us months to sort this out. However, after the initial session dealing with this memory, the energetic charge was greatly depleted, as was the case with most of Hanah's horrific memories. This meant that the body memories subsided and that the emotions associated with the memory were much less overwhelming. Hanah was far less likely to be consumed in the trauma vortex once we had processed through the memory. There was always "clean-up" involving the details, but she was never again engulfed in the body sensations and emotions as she had been before we processed the memory for the first time.

## PHASE THREE: HEALING AND DYING

By the beginning of 1995, six years into her treatment with me, new memories ceased to press for recognition. I began to see how Hanah's work with her traumatic past was becoming a transformative experience for her. She saw herself as "different," but different in a positive way. She began to see herself as knowing something that most others don't know. She viewed her history as having given her strength, and felt that all that had happened to her was significant in bringing her to this point in her life.

At one point Hanah began reading about Buddhist meditation and attended a meditation class. During one session she appeared to be embarrassed; she put her hands over her mouth before she began to speak. Finally, she told me that she already knew what she had been reading about and learning in the class. Hanah was always extremely humble; it was not like her to say something like this. Indeed, I think she already knew this information at some level; it was in her in some way. I have found in my own experience, as has Peter Levine (personal communication), that survivors of trauma often have a natural access to the spiritual world; frequently they seem to get to a spiritual level in their lives without really working at it. This was the case with Hanah.

We continued to work with memory fragments we had already processed as they intruded into Hanah's experience. The fact that parts of the memories imposed on her everyday experience meant that they were not fully processed and integrated. By now Hanah worked comfortably on a body level. She would come in, sit down, and soon begin to track her bodily experience, bringing in the other levels of her experience as well. It was much like free association anchored in the body.

As Hanah integrated more of her alters and more of the memories from her past, she began to experience profound grief. This is something I have witnessed in all trauma survivors once they get to the point of having integrated most of the traumatic material. Her grieving lasted for almost three years.

At the beginning of 1995, Hanah began to experience a series of illnesses and accidents. At the same time, her healing accelerated to the point that one day she asked me rather desperately what on earth I thought was going on. I could not answer her. She expressed concern that if she continued to get better so quickly, she would not be able to come and see me any longer. She felt that her body could not keep up with her mind, her spirit. As I reflect on this exchange now, I remind myself that we are only beginning to unravel the mystery of the mind/body correlation. I now wonder if her body (which had been exceptionally healthy all her life) simply could not keep pace with the freedom of her spirit.

Between December, 1995 and the end of 1998, Hanah was in a car accident in which she broke several ribs. She had an accident at work that resulted in a broken right arm and nerve damage to that arm. She was diagnosed with cancer and had surgery and a year of chemotherapy and radiation. A nerve problem in her left arm also required surgery. A heart problem sent her to the hospital, where she had an angiogram. Then in March of 1998, she was diagnosed with cancer again.

I don't know what to make of this, nor of the fact that at the same time she was becoming psychologically and spiritually healthier. She never was swept away in the trauma vortex between sessions. She was no longer depressed. She had given up the role of victim. She had close, loving relationships with a number of people, she could let others take care of her when it was necessary. Her alters had all integrated; the last to melt into Hanah was the Spokesperson, who spoke for so many of Hanah's "inside people" over the years. Although Hanah had expressed a wish to die and was at times suicidal, when she was diagnosed with metastatic breast cancer in August of 1995, she fought for her life. She did not understand why at the time. In retrospect, four years later, she could see that she had more healing to do, especially in her relationships with two of her children. It was as though she stayed around to complete her healing process.

Before Hanah was diagnosed the second time with cancer, she felt totally at peace most of the time. She felt that loving and being loved was all that really mattered, and was content to just be. She felt joy much of the time, and even acceptance and love for her own body, for which she had always felt such disgust and contempt. When she learned that the cancer had returned, her first reaction was anger—now that she could enjoy life, her life was threatened. In a short time she moved through this and arrived at a place where she was at peace with dying and felt that it was time for her to move on.

During the last months of her life Hanah was the happiest

she had ever been. I received a call from her one day. She said, "I am wondering why it is taking so long for me to die. I am wondering if I am just hanging around because I am having so much fun, and I suppose I don't really need to do that." She died a few weeks later.

She was adamant that her precious doll, Sweetie, would go to me. Hanah was never without Sweetie; she carried her everywhere. Sweetie was a doll made from black cloth so that "she would not get dirty." Over the years Sweetie was mended over and over again and had many new dresses. She now sits on my desk in my office, reminding me of Hanah and the resiliency of the human spirit.

# Chapter Nine

———— ·⟨⟨◉⟩⟩· ————

# MY STORY: A SURVIVOR OF INCEST AND MEDICAL ABUSE

## THE DESTRUCTION OF A SELF

I see myself walking a hospital corridor. I am wearing a hospital gown and bathrobe and carrying a set of flash cards. I read them in order: "My name is Maryanna Eckberg." "My address is 5015 Emerson Ave." "My age is twenty." "My doctor's name is Dr. Williams." "This is the University of Minnesota Hospital." "I have undergone a series of electroshock treatments." My memory fades. What did the rest of these little cards have to say to me about what had been done to me?

It seems congruent with the inhuman treatment I had suffered that this important information would be given to me in the form of little cards, with no human contact. I had just received fifty shock treatments in two and a half weeks, about three per day. I had been reduced to a state in which I did not know my own name, could not feed myself, and had lost bowel and bladder control. The treatment, ironically, was called REST—regressive electroshock therapy.

I spent four more months in the hospital regaining my capacities before I was discharged. Four months after being discharged, I returned to the university. I believe that this was my way of finding my way back to some realm of sanity. I had always known that I was smart. Perhaps I still had a brain—at least I had to attempt to prove that I did. I finished my undergraduate work, making straight As. I entered graduate school, and after the first quarter I was offered an NIMH fellowship by the chairman of the department so I could earn my Ph.D.

Achievement and overwork became my most important survival strategies. I sealed over with cement what had happened to me. I never forgot what had been done to me, but I denied its impact on my life. When each new psychotherapist I encountered over the years asked me how many shock treatments I had been given, I could not remember. I would have to go and ask the youth pastor of our church, a friend of the family, who remembered this information.

I realize now that my body had frozen in a shock organization, and that I was dissociated from my body. My diaphragm was so immobilized that I could hardly breathe. I was numb and unable to experience feelings. After this assault on my person, I did not cry for ten years. I married a man who was also estranged from his feelings; we related on an intellectual, nonfeeling level. I was very isolated, unable to allow anyone to get to know me. I had many acquaintances, but no close friends.

At twenty-nine I gave birth to my son; at thirty-one my daughter. The entry into my life of these two precious beings once again opened up my attachment system, which had been completely shut down. These years were some of the happiest of my adult life. Recent research suggests that there were not only psychological reasons for this, but biological ones as well (Henry, 1996). The hormones associated with pregnancy and nursing tend to produce a sense of well-being and calm as opposed to the adrenalized, anxious states related to trauma.

As I began to let a few people into what had been a closed system, I started to work on myself psychotherapeutically. At the outset of this endeavor, I learned how to cry; tears that had been frozen for ten years began to flow.

For the next fifteen years I lived as though I had to prove to myself that nothing unusual had happened to me. I took the attitude that if you pretend well enough you can convince, not only the world, but yourself that you are perfectly fine. I had two beautiful children and an active and successful career. I had friends; however, none of these friends was allowed access to the deeper levels of my being. Many younger women held me up as a model of a high-functioning career woman and mother. Yet beneath the surface I felt extremely anxious most of the time. I often felt overwhelmed by my feelings and by normal life events. I had panic attacks. I was hypervigilant and in almost a constant state of hyperarousal. I convinced myself that this was normal, that everyone experienced life this way.

My defensive system was impenetrable. No psychotherapist I had seen was able to get even close to exploring the traumatic incidents in my past. Not until the mid 1980s when the information on posttraumatic stress disorder found its way into the foreground of the psychological world, did I begin to see that something very extreme had happened to me and that I suffered from its effects daily. Interestingly, the long-closed door to my past was first opened by viewing a movie with my daughter. She had suggested that we see *Man Facing Southeast*. This is essentially the story of the relationship between a patient in a mental hospital and a psychiatrist, although there are many complex levels of meaning. About two-thirds of the way through, the psychiatrist decides that he must destroy the patient's truth by giving him insulin shock therapy. At this point I went into a dissociative state, in which I was living totally in my past. I thought I was crying out loud, but I was sobbing inside myself. After this, there was no way to close the door on my past. I began

193

the long journey back to integrating the painful events that I had lived through.

## THE INVESTIGATION: HOW COULD IT HAVE HAPPENED?

I was the middle child in an upper middle-class midwestern family. An exemplary "good" child, I always did what was asked of me and went out of my way to help my mother around the house. The first confusing event on the road to my personal tragedy occurred when I was twelve. I was visiting the my uncle's farm (my father's brother). A cousin, who had two children of his own, molested me several times when he could get me alone. He kissed me and fondled my breasts and genitals. Realizing that there was something very wrong about what he was doing, I went to my cousin Marilyn, my uncle's daughter. About eight years older than I was, she understood better than I did what was going on. Marilyn told her mother. But no one ever said one word to me about the incident. I was left to wonder, what did I do wrong? What did he do wrong? What were people saying about me? I learned that someone could invade my body, I could tell someone about it, but there was no help—I was on my own.

Years later when I confronted my mother about the event, she told me that my aunt had told her and my father, and that she did not know why my father never confronted the man. Four years later my father himself would be molesting me.

After this event I changed from a relatively friendly, outgoing girl into an introverted, withdrawn, shy teenager. I felt isolated with an experience that made no sense in the conservative and religious world in which I lived.

My first memory of my father sexually invading me was when I was sixteen years old. Certain pieces of my traumatic history stand out as though recorded on a photograph; this is one of them. I was standing in front of the mirror in the bathroom. My father entered the room, came up behind me, and began to fondle my breasts and genitals. He commented that I was "growing up." I froze and entered a state that I now recognize as shock. A fog of confusion gripped my mind. My father, a "pillar of the community" was wealthy, charismatic, highly respected. He could do no wrong. Yet my body recoiled at what he was doing. It felt wrong. I felt bad. I was looking at my reflection in the mirror and was feeling terrorized, confused, and ashamed. These feelings became overcoupled with my appearance, resulting in a lifelong obsession, overconcern, and even fear about how I look.

Other memories of the sexual abuse by my father are not as clear. It continued for two years, until I left home for college. It is no wonder to me now that the only two universities that interested me, California and Florida, were about as far from Minnesota as I could go and still be in the United States.

At college I attempted to dissociate the memories of the sexual abuse. I acted out by drinking, smoking, staying out late, driving recklessly, and not caring much about anything. This worked to ward off depression for a while. However, one night after we had been out drinking, I heard my dissociated voice telling my roommate about the sexual abuse by my father. After reassociating the abuse, I began the descent into depression.

During my senior year of college I dropped out of school and returned home, unable to battle the depression on my own any longer. The nightmare that was my life was just beginning.

Between 1994 and 1998 my psychotherapist, Jay, and I, in an attempt to piece together what had actually happened to me made an investigation into my history. I made a journey back to Minnesota to interview a number of people. Over the phone Jay interviewed others, whose names we obtained from my hospital records. Until 1994 I knew only the outline of what had occurred. I had been referred to a private psychiatrist, Dr. George Williams, by Bill Smith, who was the youth pastor of my family's church. I had told Dr. Williams about the incest and he obviously believed me; he broke confidentiality and spoke to Bill Smith about the sexual activity going on between me and my father. At this juncture these two men had the opportunity to intervene in an appropriate way to help me with the obvious cause of my depression—my father's violation. Unfortunately for me, neither had the integrity to do what was needed to put my life back on course. Instead of dealing with the incest, Dr. Williams put me into the hospital and began giving me electric shock therapy. The treatments began within about a week after he first saw me, three days after I entered the hospital.

After fifty shock treatments, I somehow pulled myself back together on my own, left the hospital, and returned to the university. I never questioned this strange turn of events. Why would I be given electroshock therapy? Where was my mother? How could she let this happen? What role did my father play in this? I asked none of these questions because I was afraid of disturbing my equilibrium. It took my current psychotherapist, Jay, the only psychotherapist who did not let me slip away from facing and integrating the details of my strange, violent past, to ask these questions and insist on answers.

I first looked at my hospital record in 1989 after sending for it when I was under the care of another psychiatrist. This psychiatrist did what I realize now was absolutely the wrong thing to do: He gave me the record to take home and look at by myself. When I did, I went into what I now recognize as shock. Telling no one, I put the record away for another five years. I was unable to look at it or to show it to anyone until Jay asked me to bring it to a session. Jay was shocked himself when he saw the record. In his opinion, it is the worst clinical record he has ever seen in all his years of practice.

I was admitted on April 6, 1960. Two days later regressive electroshock treatments (REST) were started. It is obvious from the nurses' notes that this treatment had been ordered when I was admitted. I was 20 years old and had experienced no prior psychotherapy or medication for my depression. Yet I was to receive a treatment reserved for chronic psychotic patients who had been hospitalized for years.

There is a short paragraph in my hospital record, scribbled in poor handwriting by somebody named Bardon. It says:

*Mental Status: Oriented. Memory ok. Affect is extremely flat and mood is depressed. There is very little personal interaction with the patient and she is obviously very withdrawn. There is evidence of much blocking and the patient appears to be operating in her own little world at times. No delusions or hallucinations were elicited. She did not appear paranoid or have ideas of reference. Limited insight. Intellectual functioning was severely bogged down. Impression: chronic undifferentiated schizophrenia.*

The record also gave the results of psychological testing. The MMPI showed "deviant ideation and depression; and also a psychopathic element which could manifest itself in sexual or other impulsive acting-out (suicide?)." But "Neither the Rorschach nor the Sentence Completion shows disorganized or autistic thinking. If deviant percepts were stimulated by the Rorschach her reality contact is firm enough to enable her to avoid verbalizing them." Yet the consensus for my diagnosis was chronic undifferentiated schizophrenia. Those doing the testing also alluded to the fact that the REST treatment plan had already been instituted, and that their results supported such a plan.

One of the questions I asked everyone when I returned to Minnesota to investigate my past was if I had ever appeared to be psychotic or to have lost contact with reality. The answer was unequivocally "no" by everyone who had known me then.

The record shows no interview with my mother. There is an

interview with my father, however, in which he states that he thinks that my preoccupation with my appearance is "sinful." He also states that he wants "patient to have shock treatments as soon as possible so that patient can go on vacation with parents to Arizona." In fact, my parents did go on vacation to Arizona. They left me alone at the hospital to be subjected to a massive assault on my brain and my person.

I knew that Dr. George Williams had died some time in the mid 1980s. My father had died in 1966. Therefore, we were unable to obtain any information from the two primary players in this incomprehensible scenario. Jay contacted the psychiatrist who is currently head of the psychiatric department at the University of Minnesota Hospital. She remembered George Williams very well. According to her, he did not favor the use of shock treatment. He was psychoanalytically oriented, well liked, and considered to be very good with students. This left Jay and me more puzzled than ever. Why would he have ordered this extreme treatment for me—a young student who had received no prior treatment for my depression.

Next Jay was able to track down a resident who had done some of the interviewing and whose name was connected to the shock treatment record. This resident gave Jay some very important information. He said that there was a study being done at the hospital at that time by a psychiatrist named Dr. Bernard Glueck. Dr. Williams had put me into the study, so that I was then under the "care" of Dr. Glueck. The resident, who is now a psychiatrist, could not remember me; I was just one of many in the study. But he expressed serious concerns about this type of psychiatric treatment and, in fact, had completely changed the direction of his work as a psychiatrist after his experience at the University of Minnesota.

This information was consistent with what I had just learned from Bill Smith, the youth pastor of my family's church. He said that when he went to the hospital to see me, he was shocked to find me on a ward with many other beds, curled up in the fetal position, unresponsive to any attempt by him to make contact with me. He told me that no one tried to interact with me; I was just given shock treatments and put back on the ward.

Jay was able to locate Bernard Glueck. His first call to Glueck resulted in Jay having to get off the phone quickly to avoid "blowing up" at this opinionated and arrogant man. After Jay explained who he was and who I was, Glueck made it clear that he believed that I had certainly been schizophrenic, and that if I were not schizophrenic now, it was because of the treatment I had received in his study. He had no reservations about the work he had done back then; he still believed that it was valid. Dr. Bernard Glueck was not the least bit interested in knowing anything about me or about how the treatment I had received in his study might have affected me over the years. He was interested only in talking about his past, the psychoanalysts he had known, and his life's work with ECT (electroconvulsive therapy), of which he was very proud.

Dr. Glueck subscribes to a complicated and bizarre theory. He believes that in persons who are psychotic or schizophrenic, the limbic system is overloaded, causing disorganization. The treatment is to depolarize the circuitry with ECT until the electriocortical waves are flattened out for up to twenty minutes. This means alpha and beta wave excitement is absent. According to Jay and to Winnicott (1943a,b) this is a kind of psychological death. Thus, if one wants to kill an internalized object or oneself, one could submit oneself to ETC.

The connection between this extreme form of treatment and psychoanalysis is apparently the idea that it makes one regress to an infantile state so one can be "reparented" as part of psychotherapeutic treatment. The state produced by regressive electric shock treatment (REST) is referred to as a regressed, childlike state, when in reality what is really being produced is an acute brain syndrome. Winnicott (1944) points out that, since one psychiatrist gives hundreds of persons ECT, he cannot see how each case could be followed up with adequate psychotherapy.

It is clear from my hospital record that I received no reparenting or psychotherapy of any kind after the shock treatments. According to Dr. Glueck, Dr. Williams had been responsible for any follow-up treatment. The nurses' notes in the record are very detailed. They mention almost no contact with Dr. Williams during or after the shock treatments.

## A BRIEF HISTORY OF
## ELECTROCONVULSIVE THERAPY (ECT)

Electroconvulsive therapy is defined as a medical procedure in which a brief electrical stimulus is used to induce a cerebral seizure for the purpose of treating specific types of mental disorders. During the 1930s four types of "somatic" (I find it ironic that somatic is the word used for these physical treatment modalities) therapies for schizophrenia were developed; three of them were insulin coma therapy, psychosurgery (prefrontal lobotomy), and pharmacological convulsive therapy. In 1938 Urgo Cerletti and Lucio Bini pioneered the fourth somatic therapy: using electric shock to induce seizures for the treatment of severe psychosis. Although they used the term electroshock, electricity was used only for to induce convulsions. They denied any effects of the electrical currents on the psychotic illness.

Convulsive therapy was originally based on the observation of a biological antagonism between epilepsy and schizophrenia. However, fifty years after it was first introduced as a treatment modality, the explanation for how it works remains a mystery. Cerletti (1940), is credited with originating ECT after witnessing electric executions of pigs at the Rome slaughterhouse. He gave the following explanation for the mechanism of ECT:

*As far as the activating mechanism is concerned I have formed this idea: electroshock violently arouses all those nervous reactions, which belong to the field of cerebral functions philogenetically organized to guard and defend life. The violent activation of the above-mentioned mechanisms has the effect of powerfully reviving, stimulating and bringing back onto an active level, all the neuro-psychism that is composed of reflex, instinctive and affective reactions which make us function well in our relationships with others, yet which lies dormant and inert in mental illnesses like schizophrenia and serious forms of depression. (Cerletti, 1950)[1]*

Although originally developed to treat schizophrenia, ECT soon became widely used for to treat major mood disorders, i.e., major depression and bipolar disorder. A typical course of ECT has always consisted of six to twelve treatments, with two to three treatments administered per week.[2]

*In the past some clinicians have used "regressive ECT," in which a prolonged and intensive course of treatment was used in order to produce a sustained delirium. The objective of this practice was to create a "regressed state" and subsequently reconstruct the patient's character. This practice has not received scientific support and as such should not be used. (Pankratz, 1980).*

When ECT was originally introduced, up to 40 percent of patients suffered complications from it, frequently compression fractures of the vertebrae. Early use of ECT was also associated with a significant mortality rate—approximately one per 1,000 patients. It is important to point out that these data are based on the typical use of ECT: a total of six to twelve treatments administered two to three times weekly, not the more extreme regime of REST to which I was subjected. A complication rate of one per 1,400 treatments has been suggested recently (Pankratz, 1980); complications include laryngospasm, prolonged apnea, prolonged seizures, tooth damage, circulatory insufficiency, cardiac arrhythmia. To this day I continue to have a cardiac arrhythmia. For many years following my exposure to ECT I had serious circulatory problems. My hands and feet were often bluish from poor circulation. At times I would become so cold that only by getting into a tub of hot water would I be able to feel warm again.

The principal adverse effect of ECT, which has been the cause of much controversy, is memory impairment. Again, it is important to point out that the research is based on the normal and moderate use of ECT (six to twelve treatments), not REST. Various types of cognitive impairment include forgetting events prior to or after the treatment, and longer lasting subjective memory loss. Although the literature on ECT, for the most part, dismisses memory loss as insignificant or nonexistent, it is also admitted that complaints of memory loss may not be completely understood and that genuine memory difficulties may not be adequately detected with available neuropsychological tests (Crowe, 1984; Zinkin, and Birtchnell, 1968). My memory of important details of my life prior to the REST treatment has been permanently lost. For instance, I have letters from friends at college but no memory of their faces or of my relationship with them. I have no memory of where I lived or what I was doing just before returning home from college. It is quite an eerie feeling to have no recollection of what I did or whom I knew.

Although claims have been made that ECT causes brain damage (Breggin, 1979), a recent comprehensive review of a large number of studies concluded that ECT—as administered today—causes no evidence of irreversible brain damage. However, the possibility remains that there may be subtle deficits which cannot be measured with currently available techniques (Weiner, 1984). I propose that ECT trauma changes the limbic system, resulting in the psychobiological effects of hypervigilance, hyperarousal, psychic numbing, avoidance, anhedonia, and feeling overwhelmed—trauma symptoms that have plagued me my entire adult life. Unfortunately, I know of no studies of ECT's impact on the neurohormonal function.

Between 1943 and 1947 D. W. Winnicott, M.D., wrote a series of letters and articles for the British Medical Journal on his concerns about "fits therapy." His points are just as compelling today. Regarding the meaning of fits therapy to the patient, he says,

> *The even course of medical evolution has been interrupted and set back, according to my view, by the treatment of mental disorder by the induction of fits—a shortcut to psychotherapy and a wonderful way of doing psychiatry without having to know anything about human nature. I do invite general practitioners to state clearly whether they favor this treatment, which has features that remind one of the more violent of the medieval attempts to drive out evil spirits.(1943)*

In addition,

> *From all this it can be seen that if a patient is asked for permission for fits therapy it is always possible that the positive answer can be, and is very likely to be, a suicidal act. That is to say, the understanding doctor might, if he knew exactly what he was doing in every individual case, offer the patient a suicidal attempt which actually does not kill. It is well known that genuine but unsuccessful attempts at suicide can have a beneficial, even curative effect, and treatment by fits could perhaps be used in this specific way.*

*But it is not so used. It tends to be used as a blunderbuss treatment with no theory to support it. (1943)*

In relation to the question of brain damage, he states,

*It is difficult to believe that physical changes, that can be relied on to do good and not to do harm, could be brought about in the brain by this blunderbuss method. I must remind members here that some doctors administer the treatment because they believe that it does damage the brain, and so cuts out irritating suppressed memories. . . . no claim is made that anyone really understands how the treatment works. (1944).*

Referring to the claim that shock therapy is given in conjunction with psychotherapy,

*I take it with a grain of salt when psychiatrists report that they give psychotherapy, using shocks only as an adjunct to the psychotherapy, unless they are contented to report having treated only a few cases. If one man has given several hundred treatments I cannot see how he has followed up each case with adequate psychotherapy. (1944).*

Clearly Winnicott was in tune with the rational reservations about so radical and violent a treatment modality. He was aware of the effect such an out-of-control experience might have for the individual patient. He remained seriously concerned with the ethical considerations of the physical treatments of mental hospital patients.

## THE STUDIES

According to Bernard Glueck himself, the study I was in at the University of Minnesota Hospital was not published. The reason for this is not clear. A perusal of published research studies turned up a number that seem almost identical. Several were authored by Glueck and his associates. Since it was something I experienced firsthand, I found it interesting and chilling to read the definition given for REST, the criteria for subjects included in the studies, and the procedure.

Regressive electroshock treatment is that method of using several electroshock treatments every day until the patient has "regressed," i.e., has reached a state of amnesia, muteness, ataxia, complete incontinence, and generally infantile behavior. These signs characterize the optimum level of acute brain syndrome associated with the electroshock therapy-induced encephalopathy. After the course of electroshock therapy, the patient can be treated with anaclitic psychotherapy. (Bonn and Boorstein, 1959)

From examples of subjects chosen for REST:

> *Difficult female schizophrenics who had been hospitalized for at least one year prior to treatment. They were all on a maximum disturbed service. Every patient had received symptomatic shock treatment and large doses of tranquilizers with little or no improvement and many had received insulin coma therapy. (Jacoby and Van Houten, 1960)*

> *104 chronic schizophrenic patients from a state hospital population served as subjects. The duration of their illnesses ranged between 3-35 years. No severe complications occurred during the treatment and recovery of these 52 experimental patients, with the exception of one death, the details of which are given in the case report [the details indicated the death was due to the treatment]. (Graber and McHugh, 1960)*

And:

> *The series of 100 cases is composed mainly of schizophrenics who had had previous adequate courses of REST and / or insulin coma therapy without lasting improvement. (Glueck, Reiss, and Bernard, 1957)*

The procedure was described by different investigators in much the same way:

> *Their object was to give electrically induced convulsions with sufficient frequency to produce a state of deep regression. They started by inducing two to three grand mal seizures daily until the desired degree of regression was reached. They considered that a patient had regressed sufficiently when he wet and soiled himself or acted and talked like a four-year-old. Their patients were confused and could not take care of their physical needs; they lost weight and frequently had to be spoon-fed. (Graber & McHugh, 1960)*

> *By the end of the first week they had difficulty in their surroundings. By the eleventh or twelfth day they usually started soiling, had to be spoon-fed and could walk only with help. At this point treatment was discontinued. (Jacoby and Van Houten, 1960)*

> *Regression is assumed to be complete when the patient manifests a majority of the following signs: There are memory loss, marked confusion, disorientation, lack of verbal spontaneity, slurring of speech to the point of complete dysarthria or muteness, and utter apathy. The patient behaves like a helpless infant, is incontinent in both bowel and bladder functions, requires spoon-feeding and, at times, tube-feeding. Frequently, he holds his food in his mouth as if unaware that he should swallow it—permitting fluids to flow out of the mouth. Neurological signs of altered cerebral function become evident toward the end of the series and indicate when treatment should be discontinued. The patient becomes progressively ataxic, until he may not be able to walk without assistance. There is*

*increased tonus with possible spastic rigidity; reflexes become more active; and, ultimately, the abnormal reflexes of Babinski and Hoffman, and sometimes ankle clonus, become evident. A grasp reflex suggestive of the frontal lobe syndrome is sometimes seen. These signs are indicative of impairment of upper motor neuron functioning. Evidence of hypothalamic, autonomic nervous system involvement is the occasional drenching sweat occurring toward the end of therapy, and the "gooseflesh" occasionally noted on the limbs and chest during treatment. After the REST ends, the patients usually continue to regress for several days, with increased apathy, rigidity, and incontinence. (Glueck, Reiss, & Bernard, 1957)*

Such description makes it difficult for me to believe that no brain damage results from such a drastic and violent treatment. In addition, regarding the motivation of doctors doing fits therapy, Winnicott says,

*Planning, if it is to be as good as jogging along, must take onto account unconscious factors. There is such a thing as a doctor's unconscious antagonism to ill people who do not respond to his therapy. In my opinion shock therapy is too violent a treatment for us to be able to make use of it, at the same time being sure that we are not unconsciously intending it to hurt the patient. (Winnicott, 1943)*

## CONCLUSIONS

After gathering the information, Jay and I had to try to make sense of it all. The subjects considered suitable for this radical treatment were seriously disturbed, persons who had been ill for years and for whom other treatments had failed. I was a college student who had been depressed for a few months and for whom no treatment of any kind had been provided. Dr. Williams, who put me into the study, did not believe in shock treatment and was known for not using it. But according to Dr. Glueck, Dr. William decided that I was a suitable subject for the study; Dr. Glueck did not screen me to determine if I was suitable. I had told Dr. Williams about the incest with my father. He was a psychoanalyst. Yet he chose not to deal with it. It is clear that he believed me, because Bill Smith, the youth pastor of the church, indicated that he did.

My hospital record is only a chart showing the dates and time of shock treatments, the anesthetic used, and the doctor who was present. There are no notes about me and how I am responding to the treatment. The interviews and test reports are poorly written and only provide support for the REST treatment. My psychotherapist has even wondered if the record was invented or forged, since the test report is not signed and the handwriting of several different persons looks similar. The only thing in the record that seems authentic are the nurses' notes. Although he was my doctor, the nurses' notes indicate that I had almost no contact with Dr. Williams all the months that I was in the hospital.

Finally, Jay could only conclude that my father had paid off the psychiatrist to "treat" me in this way so as to destroy my memory. The last thing my father would have wanted was for me to talk about our incestuous relationship. My father, who had money, influence, and charisma does show up in the hospital record, whereas my mother does not.

A number of other persons who have heard this story have independently come to the same conclusion. It took me a full year in my psychotherapy to digest this idea and to seriously consider it. Now I tend to agree. What other motivation would Dr. Williams have for such a radical decision, so unlike his typical mode of operating? Perhaps he just did not know how to handle the situation, and this was his misguided attempt to annihilate what he could not manage. I remain open to this possibility, but it seems less likely to me now than the first explanation.

It took many years for me to begin to see that Dr. Williams's role was harmful to me and protective of my father. I saw him in psychotherapy for years after I left the hospital and returned to the university, but I cannot imagine what we talked about, since we obviously could not talk about the incest and my relationship to my parents. Six years after my hospitalization, my father died. I became somewhat depressed after my father's death—a predictable occurrence, given that I carried a tremendous burden of unresolved grief, fury, and terror in relation to my father. Dr. Williams handled this by suggesting that I have more shock treatment. Fortunately, I was strong enough at this point to decline his recommendation, and I terminated treatment with him.

## THE RECONSTRUCTION OF A SELF

What does it mean to have your identity completely destroyed at age twenty? This is a question that still haunts me. I do not know anyone else who has had this experience. I still feel very isolated with it.

After being discharged from the hospital, I devoured books about the Holocaust, American Indians, slavery—all describing the destruction of the identity of individuals and of whole cultures. I think it was my way of seeking a connection to someone or something that related to my own experience.

In 1994 a colleague, who knows about my history, asked me to be the director of a center for the treatment of survivors of political torture. He said he felt that, among my other qualifications, I also knew something from my own experience about the breaking down of an individual. He helped me make a conscious connection between the experience of political torture and my own experience, even though I think I had made that connection unconsciously long ago. The politics in my case were the politics of the family, not of the state. But the objective was the same— to suppress the truth. For this reason I identify with victims of political torture, as well as victims of child abuse. Over the years, I have worked a great deal with clients from both groups. I made no conscious decision to work with these populations; people with these histories simply sought me out for treatment.

I have a photograph of the five members of my family, taken shortly after I was discharged from the hospital. My mother, father, sister, and brother appear full of energy and are smiling broadly at the camera. They seem oblivious to me. I am hunched down in the left corner of the photo looking like a constricted, trapped animal. That is exactly how I remember feeling—constricted, frozen, and trapped in a body that always felt out of control and overwhelmed with too much activation.

With sheer will power, I began to construct a posttraumatic identity. There was no room in this identity for the violinist, for the pianist, the horsewoman, or the poet. These talents and accomplishments were forgotten as all my energy went into surviving. Within four months after being discharged I was attending the university and living at home. How insane this seems to me now—to be living at home with my mother and father and to be in psychotherapy with Dr. Williams, all those who were responsible for the cruel and inhuman treatment I had received. Minds can do incredible gymnastics when necessary to incorporate incomprehensible information.

School became a refuge for me, a place of sanity, where I could earn respect. I was able to prove to myself that I still had a brain; "they" had not been able to take this away from me. In 1967 I received my Ph.D. in child and adult clinical psychology from the University of Minnesota.

For fifteen years the door to my past remained sealed shut. In 1975 I began to participate in trainings in some of the newer forms of psychotherapy. One of these was an intensive training in Gestalt therapy. In this group I was introduced to bioenergetic psychotherapy and various forms of hands-on body work (massage, cranial-sacral work, jin shin jyutsu, Rosen work). I began bioenergetic therapy and did one hands-on body work session per week. Also, I did kundalini yoga, and I saw chiropractors, osteopaths, and acupuncturists.

My rigidified, frozen body slowly began to melt. I can still recall how amazed I felt when my diaphragm became mobilized and my breathing opened up. I was able to cry. I could feel my feelings. I could sense my body. The circulatory problems disappeared. I no longer felt extremely cold.

This did not happen overnight; I would say that it took at least a year of conscientious work, during sessions and on my own at home, before appreciable changes were obvious. I continued to work on myself this way for about ten years. The core of my shock trauma—the incest and the shock treatment—remained untouched in any direct way. However, the work with my body to soften the tensions resulted in living less time in the trauma vortex and more time in a state free of hyperarousal, hypervigilance, and feeling overwhelmed.

I began to sense that I could take charge of my body to some extent, that it was not always outside my control. Yet I continued to be in massive denial about what had happened to me. I never entertained the notion that I had lived through something outside the realm of normal human experience or that the way in which I experienced myself was outside the norm. My defenses of overwork, achievement, maintaining a strong body, and always being overextended functioned well to protect me from the truth of my past.

The next chapter of my healing began by my viewing the movie *Man Facing Southeast*. A door to reassociating the pain and outrage from these drastic experiences was opened. The door was forced open a bit more a few years later, when I acquired the hospital records and looked at them for the first time. Finally I had to admit to myself that I had lived through something very extreme, which had had a shattering impact on life.

I continued to do weekly body work sessions, to see a chiropractor or an osteopath, and to see an acupuncturist. I did bioenergetic exercises at home. I was unable to find a somatic psychotherapist with whom to work, because all the somatic psychotherapists living in my area were friends and colleagues. I did some insignificant work with verbal psychotherapists. In 1989 I met Peter Levine and managed to do some intensive work with him for a number of years. In 1990 I began working with Jay, a psychoanalytically trained psychotherapist, who saw that I had not dealt directly and deeply with my traumatic past.

My dear friend and colleague, Sylvia Conant, and I had worked with each other for years using Peter Levine's method. We were attempting both to learn this method of working and to heal each other from our respective traumas. In addition, Sylvia did a body-oriented psychotherapy session with me, based on Peter Levine's model each week.

Even with all of this support, I frequently wondered how I would be able to keep functioning. My terror and anger were intense and often threatened my equilibrium. My grief was profound, and I often felt as though I would drown in it. I also experienced numerous "body memories"—sensations, often painful, that were related to the historical experience that I was working through. For instance, once my hips froze, making it very painful even to walk for months. Then I had a sciatica pain, which lasted for nine months, and following this I had a pain in my shoulder, for which I received physical therapy for months. I experienced pain in my sacrum for almost a year. In 1997 my neck became frozen so tightly that I could hardly move it from side to side. I then experienced a pain in my right foot, which lasted for three months. In all of these experiences no medical explanation for the pain was found. I treated the problems with alternative medicine (acupuncture, chiropractic), physical therapy, and Peter Levine's approach to working on a body level.

As an example of how Sylvia and I worked with these strange symptoms, I began by focusing on pain in my sacrum. I then felt as if I had too much energy in my body. I experienced tightness in my throat; my head and neck arched back as they must have done during the shock treatment. I felt spasms in my legs and feet. I entered a state of dissociation—I felt spacy and floaty. Then I focused on a squeezing sensation in my forehead, tightness in my throat, too much energy in my body. My neck and head arched again. Then I went into a dissociative state again. This was repeated several times. Finally, my legs and feet started to tremble and dis-charge energy. I felt impulses to run, to flee. I just let the energy discharge. My hands and arms began to tremble and to discharge energy, and I felt the intentional movements of wanting to push away. After a number of sessions this pattern of overcoupling, which had to do with the shock treatment experience, ceased to exist; that is the sensations that were tightly connected with each other came apart and reorganized into defensive and orienting responses.

In working through the shock treatment experience with Sylvia using Peter Levine's approach, I truly understood how painful and terrifying it had been. I experienced choking, gagging, and gasping. I felt I was being killed, yet I was unable to fight back or to escape. At least some of these responses may have been related to having been given anectine for each shock treatment, which paralyzes the skeletal muscle system, including the diaphragm. Thus, I would have had to be intubated (a breathing tube inserted through the mouth or nose into the trachea to ensure an airway) or given oxygen for each shock treatment. Because the clinical record is so poorly documented, it is not clear just what they did.

After several sessions of experiencing terror, paralysis, gasping, and choking, my body finally reorganized itself. I let out a scream of protest and outrage in which my whole body participated. I experienced the micromovements of pushing away, fight-

ing back, and running in my legs and arms, intentional movements completing after being frozen for a lifetime. My neck
thawed out, and the orienting responses returned; I was able to
move my head freely from side to side. I became aware of how
much the autonomic system was affected by the shock treatment.

As I worked with Sylvia I would experience chills, sweats,
and extreme tiredness. I also became familiar with the space I
must have been in after my mind was totally assaulted by the
shock treatments. I came to call this state "never-never land." It
is difficult to describe. I had no awareness of my body; it was like
being asleep, yet I was not asleep. It was not like any altered
state I had ever experienced. It was as though everything
stopped and I was no longer present.

To understand that this state underlies my being made it easier to understand why I have had to keep active, to keep driving
myself all my life, to feel I am in control of myself and everything
around me. Because to fall into this state is like death, yet it is
not death. Sylvia and I worked a great deal with this state, entering it and leaving it; sometimes staying in it for up to ten
minutes. A number of times this taxed Sylvia's faith in the
process. She wondered if I would emerge once again from this
strange mental state. It was very important for me to learn that
I could enter this state and then emerge, so as to feel less terror
of becoming stuck there.

We tracked through the shock treatment experience again
and again until the movements and accompanying autonomic
responses were replaced by adaptive aggressive responses.
When the incest experience intervened, we would process this
the same way, by just tracking my experience on all levels—sensations, images, behavior, emotion, and meaning.

As Sylvia and I were working on a body level to uncouple
overcoupled fragments of my traumatic past and to reassociate

pieces that do go together, Jay and I were doing something similar in my psychoanalytically oriented psychotherapy. The investigation pried apart remnants of my thinking that were linked in distorted ways and began to organize bits of information to produce a coherent picture. This did not happen without a struggle. I was in a great deal of pain. Once again, I saw how entrenched are our defenses to preserve the familiar; how frightening it is to tamper with them, even when they cause misery.

At one point I almost left therapy, having convinced myself that my therapist was inadequate. The transference is obvious now, but wasn't to me then. I had two inadequate parents; of course, at some point I would experience my therapist as inadequate. It was at a crucial time, just as we were getting to the very bottom of my traumatic past. Jay handled my attempt to squirm away well, and I continued the painful process with him.

Ordinarily, reorganizing on a cognitive level happens concurrently with reorganizing on a body level when one is doing body-oriented psychotherapy. However, I was engaged in body-oriented work with Sylvia, where there was a reorganization occurring on all levels of experience. I was also involved in a massive cognitive restructuring of my past in my work with Jay. In addition, I was seeing several different hands-on body workers. In retrospect, it all worked together in its own way.

I finally reached a point where I could talk about my history with no emotional charge. The strange pains in my body had ceased. My sense of feeling alive and wanting to be alive returned. I now have very few symptoms of posttraumatic stress disorder—the hypervigilance, hyperarousal, and feelings of being overwhelmed are largely nonexistent. I no longer overextend myself. My anxiety level is relatively normal.

After I had achieved this stabilized experience of myself, however, I had one more troubling physical symptom: I began to have difficulty swallowing. My healers and I all viewed it as yet one more somatic expression of my past trauma. It could have been the incest—oral sex. It could have been the intubation from the shock treatment. For months we speculated as the symptom worsened. Finally, I went to a doctor. I was diagnosed with a malignant tumor in the esophageal sphincter.

This experience was a powerful lesson to me. We can never know when symptoms reflect something physically wrong or something psychologically induced. It leads to another story, which I do not intend to tell here, except to mention that it is beyond my comprehension to understand why, after a lifetime of managing to avoid medical doctors, I was thrown abruptly into their arms. I don't know if I see this as a reenactment (retraumatization) or as a corrective emotional experience (this time the doctors were sincerely trying to help, and I was surrounded by loving, caring people). This question cannot be answered, I believe. However, I am alive; I am here to tell my story. This experience makes me wonder, as with Hanah's experience, if my body, which had always been so healthy, could not keep pace with my healing on other levels.

## THE EFFECT ON MY CHILDREN:
## THE TRANSGENERATIONAL EFFECTS OF TRAUMA

My two children have told me separately that the one thing that bothered them about me as they grew up was my tendency to overreact to what they perceived as minor events. They were, of course, talking about hyperarousal and feeling overwhelmed, two of the most significant symptoms of posttraumatic stress disorder. I have observed similar symptoms in them. They tend to react to situations with an excess of arousal and then to feel overwhelmed by their own excitation. They have worked very hard to learn to modulate these tendencies, with a good deal of success.

Very little is known about the transgenerational effects of trauma. It has been observed that symptoms of posttraumatic

stress disorder are passed on to children of survivors, who themselves have not experienced shock trauma. Is this passed on in
the behavior of survivors and in the atmosphere of the home? Or
does some deeper level of transmission take place that we cannot understand with our current knowledge? To me it remains a
mystery.

When each of my children became sixteen years old I told
them about my history. This was the age when the more serious
part of the trauma began for me, and I felt it important that this
information be out in the open. I told them only the bare outline
of my experience. When my daughter was nineteen years old,
she had two dreams about my traumatic past, which included
details that I had never told her. How her unconscious mind
could have had this information continues to be a mystery to me.

The first dream involved the details of how the incest began.
In her dream she is standing in the bathroom in front of the mirror. The image of herself transforms into a vision of me and then
back into a reflection of her. Her father comes in and begins to
fondle her. His image transforms back and forth between him
and an impression of my own father. She, however, reacts very
differently. In her dream she screams at her father, turns on
him, and chases him down the hall.

Her second dream involved the shock treatment experience
and was much more complex and emotional. The morning she
had the dream, Kristin called me from college and told me that
she had had a dream about my shock treatment experience and
that she now understood my pain. She said that she awoke with
her pillow wet with tears and cried for an hour after awakening.
She wrote,

*I awoke this morning crying. I was filled with pain and*
*anguish that I have never felt before. I lay there for a*
*moment sort of in a state of shock while I sifted through my*
*confusion and searched for reality. A wave of relief swept*

*over me while I realized that I had lived, really lived, a nightmare. Even after this realization, the pain remained. I fell into intense sobbing, which seemed to be my only release of this pain. It all clicked in then. I had just relived my mother's horrifying experience. Through this dream (which is definitely the most powerful and important one I've ever had), I was able to feel her pain.*

The details of her dream paralleled my shock treatment experience in an uncanny way. Like me, in the dream she was being driven to a hospital in winter; there was snow and ice on the road. She was given a drug that makes it impossible for her brain to function. She feels betrayed by her mother and other important persons in her life. At the end of her dream, she is slumped in a chair, crying hysterically. She says:

*I have been stripped of everything. They have taken my brain. I have no more creativity or motivation or will to live. I don't have anyone or anything. I don't even know who I am. What have they done to me? I sobbed harder, feeling a deep hopelessness, which I could almost see inside myself as a huge, dark, and endless hole.*

This is exactly how I felt after the shock treatment, but I had never attempted to communicate this to my daughter, nor could I have done so if I had tried. How did she know this? She ended with,

*Although this dream may seem very grim there is great beauty in it for me. It has been like a gift that I have finally received and understood after many years. I have felt something that I have been fortunate enough to miss in my life. I now understand what endless words and tears could not tell me, which is why it came through a dream. No senses were necessary for this experience—just a heart, ready to feel all of the intense emotions pouring through it.*

# Appendix

————— ❦ —————

## SOMATIC INTERVENTIONS[1]

### INDIVIDUALS

#### 1. POSITION: SEATED; SURRENDER TO OUTBREATH

Sit in a chair with both feet on the floor. When you inhale, put a little pressure on your feet. When you exhale, let up on the pressure and surrender to the exhale, making sure that you exhale all the air. Emphasis the exhale—breathing gently into the lower abdomen. Continue for a short time. You may feel some light trembling in your legs.

#### 2. POSITION: STANDING; SURRENDER TO OUTBREATH

Stand with your feet parallel and shoulder-width apart, with knees slightly bent. Place your hands on your lower abdomen and gently exhale into your hands. Make sure that you exhale all the air. Continue for a short time. You may feel some light shaking in your legs.

#### 3. POSITION: STANDING; STRESS POSITION

Stand with your feet parallel and shoulder-width apart, with your knees slightly bent. Place your fists in your lower back or your hands on your hips. Lean back slightly, making an arch with your body. As you breathe you may notice some shaking in your legs.

## 4. POSITION: STANDING; ROCKING POSE

Stand with your feet parallel and shoulder-width apart, with your knees slightly bent. Gently rock from side to side by putting all your weight on one foot, and then shift and put all your weight on the other foot. Do this very slowly.

## 5. POSITION: STANDING; HANGING OVER

Stand with your feet parallel and shoulder-width apart, with your knees slightly bent. Hang over at the waist, allowing your hands to stretch toward the floor. Your knees should be slightly bent. Your legs may begin to tremble lightly.

## 6. BALANCING ON A GYMNASTIC BALL

Sit on the gymnastic ball with legs spread slightly apart. Allow your weight to sink into the ball. Shift your weight slowly from one leg to the other. Allow yourself to play with the subtle movements of shifting and balancing. Bounce up and down very lightly. Let your bottom sink deeply into the ball.

## 7. POSITION: LYING DOWN; SURRENDER TO OUTBREATH

Lie down with your knees up and the soles of your feet on the floor. Place your hands on your lower abdomen. Exhale into your hands, surrendering to the outbreath. You may experience some light trembling in your legs.

## 8. POSITION: LYING DOWN

Lie down. Bring your knees up with the soles of your feet

on the floor. Kick vigorously until you are tired, then stop and rest. Kick again. Rest again. Do this at least three or four times.

## 9. POSITION: LYING DOWN

Lie down. Extend your legs upward. Keep extending your legs very slowly until they are almost straight, then bring them in again by bending them. Again extend them again very slowly. Do this four to five times. You may feel a slight trembling in your legs.

## 10. LYING DOWN: ROCKING POSE

Lie down. Bring your knees up and place the soles of your feet on the floor. Push and let go gently with your feet and your sacrum until you experience a gentle longitudinal (from head to feet) rocking.

## 11. POSITION: SITTING, STANDING, OR LYING DOWN

Notice how your body is organized, perhaps by becoming aware of some area of tension in your body. Now, intensify that tension. Exaggerate it very slowly and allow whatever you are experiencing to come into your awareness. Then release the exaggeration and slowly go back to where you started. Again allow what is happening into your awareness. Do this three or four times; then rest and notice your experience of yourself.

## PAIRS

## 1. POSITION: LYING DOWN; HOLDING HEAD

The client lies down. The therapist sits above the client's head, slips his hands under the occipital area of the head, and gently lifts the head off the floor about an inch. Hold the client's head like this for ten to fifteen minutes. A variation is to gently move the client's head from side to side or up and down.

## 2. POSITION: STANDING; HAND PUSH

The therapist stands in a martial arts stance facing the client, with right hands together. The client then pushes and the therapist offers resistance with her hand. Invite the client to gradually increase the pressure, and increase your resistance as well. Be sure to sense and move from your center and to sense your own power. After you have finished with the right arm, move to the left arm, then do this with both arms. The client should be sure to communicate how much pressure he wants as resistance.

## 3. POSITION: STANDING; BACK TO BACK PUSH

Stand with your back touching the client's back. The client then walks backward, pushing you forward. It is important for the client to sense her center and power while doing this. The client should communicate how much resistance she wants.

## 4. POSITION: STANDING

The therapist and client hold hands and lean back with knees bent. Slowly descend to a squatting position, maintaining your balance by leaning back and pulling on your partner's hands. Then slowly rise to a standing position. Go up and down slowly three or four times.

## 5. POSITION: LYING DOWN

The client lies down on his back with knees bent. The therapist places a pillow on his shoulder. The client places one foot at a time on the pillow and extends his leg slowly. The purpose is for the client to connect to his center and strength. The therapist simply resists and does not push back. Do this several times with each leg.

## 6. POSITION: LYING DOWN; LOWER BACK SUPPORT

The client is lying down. The therapist places her hand and forearm under the client's lower back. The client's back will slowly drop into the therapist's hands. After a few minutes the therapist asks if it is okay to place her hand on the client's abdomen. If the client gives permission, the therapist places her other hand on the client's abdomen.

## GROUP

All of the somatic interventions listed for individuals and pairs can be done in a group. In addition, the following interventions may be used with a group.

## 1. HEALING CIRCLE.

All are seated or lying down on the floor. One person is in the center surrounded by the rest of the group. Each person places one hand on the person in the center and one hand on the person next to him. Breathe freely and focus on sending and receiving energy.

## 2. MASSAGE CIRCLE.

Stand with everyone facing in the same direction. Massage the neck and shoulders of the person in front of you slowly and firmly, breathing openly as you do so.

## 3. MANDALA HEART CIRCLE.

Everyone lies down with her head facing toward the center. Hold hands with the person next to you. Focus your attention on your chest area. Exaggerate the tension in your chest and release it. Do this three or four times.

Reach your chest toward the ceiling so that your back lifts slightly off the floor. Then let your chest drop. Do this about three times. Breathe normally and notice the sensations in the area of your heart. Lightly squeeze the hands of the person next to you and again notice the sensations in the area of your heart. What are you feeling? Can you put words to the sensations and feelings? What is your heart saying?

4. STAND HOLDING HANDS.

Raise your hands upward and back so that your body makes a slight arch backwards. Bend your knees and breathe deeply.

5. EVERYONE LIES DOWN WITH HIS HEAD FACING TOWARD THE CENTER.

Hold hands. Your feet should be about two feet apart. Stretch into your right heel, extending the right leg downward. Then release and stretch into your left heel, extending the left leg downward. Stretch into the right heel again, and so on. There should be a rotating motion in the pelvis as each leg extends and then releases.

# Chapter Notes

———— ⦿ ————

## CHAPTER ONE

1. See Boyd, Blow, and Orgain, 1993; Cottler et al., 1992; Groth, 1979; Henry, 1996; Herman, 1992; Krystal, 1988; Levi, 1988; Pennebaker, 1993; Pribor et al., 1993; Putman, 1989; Saxe et al., 1994; Schmitt and Nocks, 1984; Seghorn, Boucher, and Pentky, 1987; Soumi, 1994; Spiegal, 1992; van der Kolk, 1987, 1989, 1994, 1996; van der Kolk and van der Hart, 1989, 1995; van der Kolk and Fisler, 1995; van der Kolk et. al., 1993.

2. van der Kolk, Perry, and Herman, 1991; Herman, 1992; Boyd, Blow, and Orgain, 1993; Cottler et al., 1992; Schmitt and Nocks, 1984.

3. "Los desaparecidos" (the disappeared) refers to thousands of persons in Central and South American countries who were arrested and then disappeared without a trace. It is known that they were tortured and killed.

4. See Levine (1991, 1997) for a comprehensive review of these symptoms.

5. Timerman, (1988), *Prisoner Without a Name, Cell Without*

*a Number.* p. 34. Timerman was a victim of political torture in Argentina during the "dirty war."

6. van der Kolk, 1987, 1995, 1996; van der Kolk and van der Hart, 1991; Siegel, 1993.

CHAPTER TWO

1. For a definition of the "disappeared" see Chapter One, note 3.

2. See van der Kolk, 1997, 1989, 1994, 1996; van der Kolk and van der Hart, 1989, 1995; van der Kolk and Fisler, 1995; Siegel, 1993; Schacter, 1987.

3. Goodman and Teicher, 1988; Hilton, 1997; Smith, Clauce, and Imes, 1998; Hunter and Struve, 1998.

CHAPTER THREE

1. The terms transference and countertransference are used to refer to all feelings that the client and therapist bring to the clinical relationship (Stolorow, Atwood and Brandschaft, 1994).

2. Herman, 1992; van der Kolk, 1996; Wilson and Lindy, 1994.

3. Danieli, 1994; Figley, 1995; Herman, 1992; McCann and Pearlman, 1990; Pearlman and Saakvitne, 1994; van der Kolk, 1994, 1996.

CHAPTER FOUR

1. References related to this topic could fill pages. Some of primary interest are: Reich, 1970; Becker,1975; Kohlberg,1983,1984.

2. There are fourteen *departmentos* in El Salvador (similar to states in the U.S.) A well-known joke in El Salvador is: How many *departmentos* are there in El Sal-

vador? Eleven, because La Paz (peace), La Libertad (liberty), and La Unión (union) don't exist.

3. From *An Interrupted Life: The Diaries of Etty Hillesum 1941–43*. (New York: Pantheon Books, 1983), p. 247.

CHAPTER FIVE

1. On one wall of the salon hung a large portrait of Ignacio Martín Baró, one of the six Jesuit priests assassinated on this university campus in 1989. It felt moving and appropriate to have him in the room with us.

2. Armed illegal groups continue to act, unknown individuals continue to execute innocent people, and military weapons are freely used, without fear of reprisal. See "La Voz: The Monthly Magazine of the El Salvador Human Rights Commission" 3, no. 34 (1995).

CHAPTER SEVEN

1. Jean Améry was an Austrian philosopher who was tortured by the Gestapo because he was active in the Belgian resistance, and then deported to Auschwitz because he was Jewish. Quoted in P. Levi, *The Drowned and the Saved*. (New York: Vintage Books, 1989), p. 25.

2. The Healing Center for Survivors of Political Torture was founded by Don Johnson and myself with a seed grant from the United Nations.

CHAPTER NINE

1. Milligan, 1946; Cerletti, 1950; Lowenbach, 1943; Kalinowsky and Hoch, 1946.

2. Crowe, 1984; Kalinowsky and Hoch, 1946; Lowenbach, 1943.

APPENDIX

1. Most of these interventions come from the area of bioenergetics or from the work of Stanley Keleman.

# References

Ahsen, A. (1973). *Basic Concepts in Eidetic Psychotherapy.* New York: Brandon House Press.

Becker, E. (1975). *Escape from Evil.* New York: The Free Press.

Bonn, E. M., & Boorstein, S. (1959). Regressive electroshock therapy and anaclitic psychotherapy. A case report. *Menninger Clinic Bulletin,* 23, 190–201.

Boyd, C. J., Blow, F., & Orgain, L. S. (1993). Gender differences among African-American substance abusers. *Journal of Psychoactive Drugs*, 25 (4), 301–5.

Breggin, P. R. (1979). *Electroshock: Its Brain Disabling Effects.* New York: Springer Publishing Co.

Briere, J. (1988). Long-term clinical correlates of childhood sexual victimization. *Annals of the New York Academy of Science,* 528, 327–334.

Caruth, C. (Ed.). (1995). *Trauma: Explorations in Memory.* London: Johns Hopkins University Press.

Cerletti, U. (1950). Old and new information about electroshock. *American Journal of Psychiatry,* 107, 87–93.

Conger, J. P. (1988). *Jung & Reich: The Body as Shadow.* Berkeley, CA: North Atlantic Books.

Conger, J. P. (1994). *The Body in Recovery: Somatic Psychotherapy and the Self.* Berkeley, CA: North Atlantic Books.

Cottler, E. B., Comptom, W. M., Madager, D., Spitzaagel, E. L., & Jasca, A. (1992). Posttraumatic stress disorder among substance users from the general population. *American Journal of Psychiatry,* 149, (5), 664–675.

Crowe, R. R. (1984). Electroconvulsive therapy: a current perspective. *New England Journal of Medicine,* 114, 973–988.

Danieli, Y. (1994). Countertransference and trauma: Self healing and training issues. In M. B. Williams & J. F. Sommer (Eds.), *Handbook of Posttraumatic Therapy.* Westport, CT.: Greenwood Press.

Eckberg, M. (1997a). A psychologist in El Salvador. *Bioenergetic Analysis: The Clinical Journal of the International Institute for Bioenergetic Analysis,* 8 (1), 28–42.

Eckberg, M. (1997b) A psychologist in El Salvador, Part II. *Somatics Magazine-Journal of the Mind / Body Arts and Sciences,* 11 (2), 26–33 & (1977) *Bioenergetic Analysis: The Clinical Journal of the International Institute for Bioenergetic Analysis,* 8 (1), 43–57.

European Association for Body-oriented Psychotherapy. (1995). EABP Secretariat, Geneva, Switzerland.

Figley, C. G. (Ed.). (1995). *Compassion Fatigue: Coping with Secondary Stress Disorder in Those Who Treat the Traumatized.* New York: Brunner/Mazel.

Fink, D. L. (1988). The core self: A developmental perspective on the dissociative disorders. *Dissociation,* 1 (1), 43–47.

Glueck, B. C. (1957). Session on psychiatry; regressive shock therapy. *American Journal of Occupational Therapy,* 8–11. 217–219.

Glueck, B. C., Reiss, H., & Bernard, L. E. (1957). Regressive electric shock therapy—preliminary report on 100 cases. *Psychiatric Quarterly,* 31, 117–136.

Goodman, M., & Teicher, A. (1988). To touch or not to touch. *Psychotherapy,* 25 (Winter), no. 4.

Graber, H. K., & McHugh, R. B. (1960). Regressive electroshock therapy in chronic schizophrenia, a controlled study. Preliminary report. *Lancet,* 80, 24–27.

Groth, A. N. (1979). Sexual trauma in the life histories of sex offenders. *Victimology,* 4, 6–10.

Henry, J. (Feb. 29–Mar. 4, 1996). Dissociation, alexithymia secondary to trauma and disrupted attachment. *2nd Annual Conference on Trauma, Loss, and Dissociation,* Alexandria, VA.

Herman, J. (1992). *Trauma and Recovery.* New York: Basic Books.

Hilton, R. (1997). *Touching in Psychotherapy: Therapists at Risk.* New Jersey: Jason Aronson.

Hunter, M., & Struve, J. (1998). *The Ethical Use of Touch in Psychotherapy.* CA: Sage Publications.

Jacoby, M. G., & Babikian, H. M. (1973). Regressive shock therapy. *American Journal of Psychiatry,* 130, 269–273.

Jacoby, M. G., & Van Houten, Z. (1960). Regressive shock therapy. *Diseases of the Nervous System,* 21, 582–583.

Johnson, D. A. (1996). Testimony before the House Committee

on International Relations Subcommittee on International Operations and Human Rights.

Kalinowsky, L. B. ,& Hoch, P. H. (1946). *Shock Treatment and Other Somatic Procedures in Psychiatry*. New York: Grune & Stratton.

Kardiner, A. (1941). *The Traumatic Neuroses of War.* New York: Hoeber.

Keleman, S. (1975a). *The Human Ground, Sexuality, Self and Survival*. Berkeley, CA: Center Press.

Keleman, S. (1975b). *Your Body Speaks its Mind*. Berkeley, CA: Center Press.

Keleman, S. (1979). *Somatic Reality*. Berkeley, CA: Center Press.

Keleman, S. (1985). *Emotional Anatomy*. Berkeley, CA: Center Press.

Kohlberg, L. (1983). *The Philosophy of Moral Development*. New York: Harper & Row.

Kohlberg, L. (1984). *The Psychology of Moral Development*. New York: Harper & Row.

Krystal, H. (1988). *Integration and Self-Healing: Affect, Trauma, and Alexithymia*. Hillsdale, NJ: Analytic Press.

Levi, P. (1988). *The Drowned and the Saved*. New York: Summit Books, 72–73.

Levine, P. (1991).The body as healer: A revisioning of trauma and anxiety. *Somatics*, 13 ( l), 18–27.

Levine, P. (1997). *Waking the Tiger: Healing Trauma*. Berkeley, CA: North Atlantic Books.

Lewis, D. O. & Balla, D. (1976). *Delinquency and Psychopathology*. New York: Grune & Stratton.

Lewis, D. O., Shanok, S. S., Pincus, J. H., & Glaser, G. H. (1979). Violent juvenile delinquency: Psychiatric, neurological, psychological, and abuse factors. *Journal of the American Academy of Child Psychiatry,* 18, 307–319.

Lowen, A. (1958). *The Language of the Body*. New York: Collier Books.

Lowen, A. (1972). *Depression and the Body*. New York: Coward–McCann.

Lowen, A. (1965). *Love and Orgasm*. New York: Signet Books.

Lowen, A. (1975). *Bioenergetics*. New York: Coward–McCann.

Lowenbach, H. (1943). Electric shock treatment of mental disorders. *No. Carolina Medical Journal,* 4, 123–125.

McCann, I. L., & Pearlman, L. A. (1990). Vicarious traumatization: A framework for understanding the psychological effects of working with victims. *Journal of Traumatic Stress,* 3, 131–149.

McNaughten, I. (1996). *Minding the Body; Embodying the Mind*. Private publication. Vancouver, Canada: Bodynamic Institute.

Miller, P. (1998). Healing the wounded. *Yoga Journal,* 138 (January/February), 20–25.

Milligan, W. L. (1946). Psychoneurosis treated with electrical convulsions, intensive method. *Lancet,* 2, 516–520.

Pankratz, W. J. (1980). Electroconvulsive therapy: The position of the Canadian Psychiatric Association. *Canadian Journal of Psychiatry,* 25(6), 509–514.

Pattison, E. M., & Kahan, J. (1983). The deliberate self-harm syndrome. *American Journal of Psychiatry,* 140, 867–872.

Pearlman, L. A. and Saakvitne, K. W. (1994). *Trauma and the Therapist: Countertransference and Vicarious Traumatization in Psychotherapy with Incest Survivors.* New York: W.W. Norton.

Pennebaker, J. W. (1993). Putting stress into words: Health, Linguistic, and therapeutic implications. *Behavior Research and Therapy,* 31 (6), 539–548.

Pert, C. (1995). Emotions and the mind/body connection. *First Annual Alternative Therapy Symposium,* San Diego, CA.

Pierrakos, J. (1973) Series of papers on corenergetics. New York: Institute for the New Age.

Pierrakos, J. (1987). *Corenergetics: Developing the Capacity to Love and Heal.* Mendocino, CA: Life Rhythm Publications.

Pribor, E. F., Yutzy, S. H., Dean, T., & Wetzel, R. D. (1993). Briquet's syndrome, dissociation, and abuse. *American Journal of Psychiatry,* 150, 1507–1511.

Putnum, F. W. (1989). *Diagnosis and Treatment of Multiple Personality Disorder.* New York: Guilford.

Reich, W. (1961a). *Character Analysis.* New York: Noonday Press.

Reich, W. (1961b). *The Function of the Orgasm.* New York: Noonday Press.

Reich, W. (1970). *The Mass Psychology of Fascism.* New York: Farrar, Straus, & Giroux.

Saxe, G. N., Chinman, G., Berkowitz, R., Hall, K., Lieberg, G., Schwartz, J., & van der Kolk, B. A. (1994). Somatization in patients with dissociative disorders. *American Journal of Psychiatry,* 151, 1329–1335.

Schacter, D. (1987). Implicit memory: History and current status. *Journal of Experimental Psychology: Learning Memory, and Cognition,* 13, 501–18.

Schmitt, J. M., & Nocks, J. J. (1984). Alcoholism treatment of Vietnam veterans with posttraumatic stress disorder. *Journal of Substance Abuse Treatment,* 1 (3),179–89.

Seghorn, T. K., Boucher, R. J., & Prentky, R. A. (1987). Childhood sexual abuse in the lives of sexually aggressive offenders. *Journal of the American Academy of Child and Adolescent Psychiatry,* 26, 262–67.

Siegel, D. (April 15–18, 1993) Memory, trauma, and flashbacks. 6th Annual Western Clinical Conference on Multiple Personality Disorder and Dissociation, Irvine, CA.

Smith, E. W., Clance, P. R., and Imes, S. (1998). *Touch in Psychotherapy.* New York: Guilford Press.

Soumi, S. (Feb. 29–Mar. 4, 1996). Trauma, attachment and state modulation dynamics in primates. 2nd Annual Conference on Trauma, Loss, and Dissociation, Alexandria, VA.

Spiegel, D. (1992). Effects of psychosocial support on patients with metastatic breast cancer. *Journal of Psychosocial Oncology,* 10, 113–120.

Squire, L. R. (1994). Declarative and nondeclarative memory; Multiple brain systems supporting learning and memory. In D. L. Schacter & E. Tulving (Eds.), *Memory Systems.* Cambridge, MA.: MIT Press.

Stolorow, R., Atwood, G., & Brandchaft, B. (1994). *The Intersubjective Perspective.* Northvale, NJ: Jason Aronson.

Terr, L. C. (1979). Children of Chowchilla: A study of psychic trauma. *Psychoanalytic Study of the Child,* 34, 552–623.

Terr, L. C. (1983). Chowchilla revisited: The effects of psychic trauma four years after a school-bus kidnapping. *American Journal of Psychiatry,* 140, 1543–1550.

Terr, L. C. (1993). *Unchained Memories.* New York: Basic Books.

Timerman, J. (1988). *Prisoner Without a Name, Cell Without a Number.* New York: Vintage Books.

van der Kolk, B. A. (1987). *Psychological Trauma.* Washington, DC: American Psychiatric Press, Inc.

van der Kolk, B. A. (1989). The compulsion to repeat the trauma: Revictimization, attachment and masochism. *Psychiatric Clinics of North America,* 12, 389–411.

van der Kolk, B. A. (1994). The body keeps the score: Memory and the evolving psychobiology of posttraumatic stress. *Harvard Review of Psychiatry,* 1, (5), 253–65.

van der Kolk, B. A. (1996). *Traumatic Stress: The Effects of Overwhelming Experience on Mind, Body, and Society.* New York: Guilford Press.

van der Kolk, B. A. & van der Hart, O. (1989). Pierre Janet and the breakdown of adaptation in psychological trauma. *American Journal of Psychiatry,* 146, 1530–1540.

van der Kolk, B. A., & Fisler, R. (1995). Dissociation and the fragmentary nature of traumatic memories: Review and experimental confirmation. *Journal of Traumatic Stress,* 8 (4), 505–525.

van der Kolk, B. A., Perry, J. C., & Herman, J. L. (1991). Childhood origins of self-destructive behavior. *American Journal of Psychiatry,* 148 (12), 1665–1671.

van der Kolk, B. A., Roth, S., Pelcovitz, D., & Mandel, F. S. (1993). *Complex PTSD: Results of the PTSD Field Trials for DSM–IV.* Washington, DC: American Psychiatric Association.

van der Kolk, B. A., & van der Hart, O. (1995). The intrusive past: The flexibility of memory and the engraving of trauma. In Caruth, C. (Ed.), *Trauma: Explorations in Memory.* London: Johns Hopkins University Press.

Vesti, P., & Kastrup, M. (1995). Refugee status, torture, and adjustment. In Freedy, J. R. & Hobfoll, S. E. (Eds.), *Traumatic Stress: From Theory to Practice.* New York: Plenum Press, 213–233.

Weiner, R. J. (1984). Does electroconvulsive therapy cause brain damage? *The Behavioral and Brain Sciences,* 7, 1–53.

Whitfield, C. L. (1995). *Memory and Abuse: Remembering and Healing the Effects of Trauma.* Florida: Health Communications, Inc.

Wilson, J., & Lindy, J. (1994). *Countertransference in the Treatment of PTSD.* New York: Guilford.

Winnicott, D.W. (1943a). Shock treatment of mental disorder. Letter to *British Medical Journal.*

Winnicottt, D.W. (1943b). Treatment of mental disease by induction of fits. Letter to *British Medical Journal.*

Winnicott, D.W. (1944a). Introduction to a symposium on the psycho-analytic contribution to the theory of shock therapy. Read at the British Psycho-Analytic Society, 15 March, 1944.

Winnicott, D.W. (1944b). Shock therapy. Letter to *British Medical Journal.*

Winnicott, D.W. (1947). Physical therapy of mental disorder. *British Medical Journal,* 17 May, 1947.

REFERENCES

Zinkin, S., & Birtchnell, J. (1968). Unilateral electroconvulsive therapy: Its effects on memory and its therapeutic efficacy. *British Journal of Psychiatry,* 114, 973–988.

# Index

ABOUT THE AUTHOR

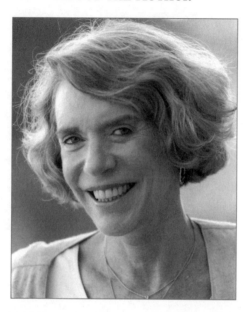

Maryanna Eckberg devoted her career to helping trauma victims and the victims of political torture. Born in Minnesota, she received a doctorate in child and clinical psychology from the University of Minnesota in 1967. In 1975 in Minnesota she began to train in gestalt and bioenergetic therapy, and started a ten-year process of training with Stanley Keleman. In 1979 Dr. Eckberg became a certified bioenergetic therapist, and then a trainer for the Bioenergetic Society of Northern California. A faculty member at California Institute of Integral Studies in San Francisco, she directed the Clement Street Counseling Center and co-founded the Healing Center for the Survivors of Political Torture with Don Hanlon Johnson in 1996. She worked for many years in El Salvador with the Commission on Human Rights, and at the Universidad José Simeón Cañas. Her work during the last years of her life focused on publishing and speaking on somatic and verbal interventions in the treatment of posttraumatic stress disorder. She died in October, 1999.